Investigating Sch‹

MW01286151

Investigating School Psychology provides a fascinating exploration of the field of school psychology through the lens of pseudoscience and fringe science. Contributions from leaders in the fields of school psychology, clinical psychology, and education honor the role of science in psychology while also exploring and guarding against the harms that pseudoscience can cause.

School psychology and, more broadly, the field of education are particularly susceptible to pseudoscience, fads, and maintaining the status quo by resisting the adoption of new ideas. Using an exhaustive review of the current literature, this book discusses various concepts in school psychology that have been largely discredited and many practices that continue to exist with little to no scientific support. Each chapter helps differentiate between dubious and evidence-based approaches while providing a useful resource for practicing school psychologists and educators to distinguish between science and pseudoscience in their everyday work. The book's discussion of the harmful nature of pseudoscience in school psychology is inclusive of all students, such as students with disabilities, those diagnosed with neurodevelopmental disorders, those with academic problems, and all other children in schools.

Investigating School Psychology is valuable supplemental reading in undergraduate and graduate courses in education and school psychology and is also a beneficial reference for practicing school psychologists to distinguish between science and pseudoscience in their practice.

Michael I. Axelrod, PhD, is the Director of the Human Development Center and a Professor in the Department of Psychology at the University of Wisconsin–Eau Claire, USA. He is a Nationally Certified School Psychologist and Licensed Psychologist. His published books include *Behavior Analysis for School Psychologist, School-Based Behavioral Intervention Case Studies: Effective Problem Solving for School Psychologists,* and *Reading Intervention Case Studies for School Psychologists.*

Stephen Hupp, PhD, is a Licensed Clinical Psychologist and Professor of Psychology at Southern Illinois University Edwardsville (SIUE), USA. In 2015, he won the Great Teacher Award from the SIUE Alumni Association. He is the editor of *Skeptical Inquirer* magazine, and he has published several books including *Pseudoscience in Therapy* and *Great Myths of Child Development.*

Investigating Psychology Pseudoscience

Series Editor

Stephen Hupp, PhD, is a Clinical Psychologist and Professor of Psychology at Southern Illinois University Edwardsville (SIUE) in the United States. In 2015, he won the Great Teacher Award from the SIUE Alumni Association. He has published several books including *Pseudoscience in Therapy* and *Dr. Huckleberry's True or Malarkey? Superhuman Abilities*.

The science of psychology has continued to grow exponentially over the last century. Unfortunately, pseudoscience in psychology has grown at an even faster pace, and yet very few texts have a primary emphasis on pseudoscience, fringe science, or other controversial topics in psychology.

The *Investigating Psychology Pseudoscience* series offers a fresh look into topics that have commonly been characterized as pseudoscience. The series considers early research while also incorporating the latest investigations into controversial topics. Scientific investigations into the fringe aspects of psychology can often reveal scientific principles, identify alternative explanations, and highlight the many ways the human brain can be deceived. These books are designed to help students, academics, professionals, and everyone else consider the full range of investigations that contribute to psychological science, pseudoscience, and everything in between.

Books in the Series

Investigating Clinical Psychology
Pseudoscience, Fringe Science, and Controversies
Jonathan N. Stea and Stephen Hupp

Investigating School Psychology
Pseudoscience, Fringe Science, and Controversies
Michael I. Axelrod and Stephen Hupp

For more information, please refer to www.routledge.com/Series+Investigating+Psychology/book-series/IPP

Investigating School Psychology

Pseudoscience, Fringe Science, and Controversies

Edited by Michael I. Axelrod and Stephen Hupp

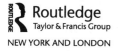

Routledge
Taylor & Francis Group

NEW YORK AND LONDON

Cover image: Getty Images © fcafotodigital and subjug

First published 2024
by Routledge
605 Third Avenue, New York, NY 10158

and by Routledge
4 Park Square, Milton Park, Abingdon, Oxon, OX14 4RN

Routledge is an imprint of the Taylor & Francis Group, an informa business

Library of Congress Cataloguing-in-Publication Data
Names: Axelrod, Michael I., editor. | Hupp, Stephen, editor.
Title: Investigating school psychology : pseudoscience, fringe science, and controversies / edited by Michael I. Axelrod and Stephen Hupp.
Description: New York, NY : Routledge, 2024. | Series: Investigating psychology pseudoscience | Includes bibliographical references and index.
Identifiers: LCCN 2023056648 (print) | LCCN 2023056649 (ebook) | ISBN 9781032209760 (paperback) | ISBN 9781032209746 (hardback) | ISBN 9781003266181 (ebook)
Subjects: LCSH: School psychology. | School mental health services. | Educational psychology. | Pseudoscience.
Classification: LCC LB1027.55 .I58 2024 (print) | LCC LB1027.55 (ebook) | DDC 370.15--dc23/eng/20240110
LC record available at https://lccn.loc.gov/2023056648
LC ebook record available at https://lccn.loc.gov/2023056649

ISBN: 978-1-032-20974-6 (hbk)
ISBN: 978-1-032-20976-0 (pbk)
ISBN: 978-1-003-26618-1 (ebk)

DOI: 10.4324/9781003266181

Typeset in Sabon
by MPS Limited, Dehradun

For my students (M.I.A)

For the Committee for Skeptical Inquiry, publisher of *Skeptical Inquirer: The Magazine for Science and Reason* (S.H.)

Contents

Other Books

Other Books in This Series

- *Investigating Pop Psychology*
- *Investigating Clinical Psychology*
- And more to come

Other Books by Michael I. Axelrod

- *Reading Intervention Case Studies for School Psychologists*
- *School-Based Behavioral Intervention Case Studies*
- *Behavior Analysis for School Psychologists*
- *Great Myths of Adolescence*

Other Books by Stephen Hupp

- *Science-Based Therapy: Raising the Bar for Emprically Supported Treatments*
- *Pseudoscience in Therapy: A Skeptical Field Guide*
- *Pseudoscience in Child and Adolescent Psychotherapy: A Skeptical Field Guide*
- *Child and Adolescent Psychotherapy: Components of Evidence-Based Treatments for Youth and their Parents*
- *Great Myths of Child Development*
- *Great Myths of Adolescence*
- *Thinking Critically about Child Development: Examining Myths and Misunderstandings*
- *Dr. Huckleberry's True or Malarkey? Superhuman Abilities: Game Book for Skeptical Folk*

Contributors

Audrey Ambrosio, BA, is a Doctoral Student in the Clinical Psychology program at the University of Southern Mississippi.

Michael I. Axelrod, PhD, is a School Psychologist, the Director of the Human Development Center, and a Professor of Psychology at University of Wisconsin–Eau Claire.

Parker S. Beckman, BS, is a Doctoral Student in the School Psychology program at Indiana University–Bloomington, USA.

John C. Begeny, PhD, is the Founder of Helps Education Fund and a Professor of Psychology at North Carolina State University, USA.

Scott Bellini, PhD, is a Licensed Psychologist, the Director of the Social Skills Research Clinic at the Institute for Child Study, and an Associate Professor of School Psychology at Indiana University–Bloomington, USA.

Nicholas F. Benson, PhD, is a Nationally Certified School Psychologist, Licensed Psychologist, Associate Professor, and Director of the School Psychology Program at Baylor University.

Matthew K. Burns, PhD, is the Fein Professor of Special Education at the University of Florida, USA.

Angela Capuano, PhD, BCAB-D, is a Clinical Psychologist, Board Certified Behavior Analyst-Doctoral, and Adjunct Lecturer of Applied Behavior Analysis at the University of Michigan–Dearborn, USA.

Sarah J. Conoyer, PhD, is a School Psychologist and an Associate Professor of Psychology at Southern Illinois University Edwardsville, USA.

Emily R. DeFouw, PhD, BCBA, is an Assistant Professor of School Psychology at the University of Southern Mississippi, USA.

Arianna Delgadillo, BS, is a Doctoral Student in the Clinical Psychology program at the University of Southern Mississippi, USA.

Lauren E. Delgaty, MA, is a Doctoral Student in the School Psychology program in the School of Education at the University of North Carolina at Chapel Hill, USA.

Stefan C. Dombrowski, PhD, is a Licensed Psychologist and Professor and Director of the School Psychology Program at Rider University, Lawrenceville, NJ, USA.

Lauren Erp, MA, is a Doctoral Student in the Clinical Psychology program at the University of Southern Mississippi, USA.

Ryan L. Famer, PhD, is the Director of the Psychological Services Center, Director of the Educational Specialist program in School Psychology, and a Clinical Assistant Professor at The University of Memphis.

Angela Fontanini-Axelrod, PhD, is a Nationally Certified School Psychologist, Licensed School Psychologist, and Assistant Professor of School Psychology at the University of Wisconsin–Stout.

Jamie Haas, BA, graduated from Southern Illinois University Edwardsville, USA.

Rahma M. Hida, PhD, is an Attending Psychologist at Boston Children's Hospital and Instructor of Psychology at Harvard Medical School, USA.

Stephen Hupp, PhD, is a Professor of Psychology at Southern Illinois University Edwardsville. He is also the editor of *Skeptical Inquirer: The Magazine for Science and Reason.*

Sara Jordan, PhD, is a Professor and Director of the School of Psychology and is affiliated with the Clinical Psychology doctoral program at the University of Southern Mississippi.

Samantha Kesselring, MA, PMLHP, is a School Psychology doctoral candidate at the University of Nebraska–Lincoln.

Kim Killu, PhD, BCBA-D, is a Limited License Psychologist, Board Certified Behavior Analyst-Doctoral, and Professor of Applied Behavior Analysis and Special Education at the University of Michigan–Dearborn.

Chad E. L. Kinney, PhD, BCBA-D, is a Behavior Analyst and an Assistant Professor of Psychology & Counseling at Georgian Court University.

Maddison Knott, BS, is a Doctoral Student in the Clinical Psychology program at the University of Southern Mississippi.

Zachary C. LaBrot, PhD, is a Licensed Psychologist and an Assistant Professor of School Psychology at the University of Southern Mississippi, USA.

Hanna S. Lim, BS, is a Doctoral Student in the School Psychology program at Indiana University–Bloomington.

Kathrin E. Maki, PhD, is a School Psychologist and an Assistant Professor of School Psychology at the University of Florida.

Marisa E. Marraccini, PhD, is an Assistant Professor of School Psychology in the School of Education at the University of North Carolina at Chapel Hill.

Jeremy Miciak, PhD, is an Associate Research Professor at the University of Houston and affiliated faculty with the Texas Institute for Measurement, Evaluation, and Statistics (TIMES) and the Texas Center for Learning Disorders.

Telieha J. Middleton is a Research Assistant in the School of Education at the University of North Carolina at Chapel Hill.

Avalon S. Moore, BA, is a Postgraduate Research Associate in the Yale OCD Research Clinic within the Department of Psychiatry at The Yale School of Medicine.

Emilea Rejman, MSc, is a School Psychology Doctoral Student at the University of Nebraska–Lincoln.

Susan M. Swearer, PhD, LP, is the Willa Cather Professor of School Psychology and Chair of the Department of Educational Psychology at the University of Nebraska–Lincoln.

Amanda M. VanDerHeyden, PhD, is the President of Education Research & Consulting in Alabama and Founder of SpringMath (www. springmath.com). Her full biography can be found here: https://www. springmath.org/amanda-vanderheyden.

Bertha Vazquez, MS, is the Education Director of The Center for Inquiry which currently includes three projects, The Teacher Institute for Evolutionary Science (TIES), ScienceSaves, and Generation Skeptics. She is also the editor and contributing author of the book, *On Teaching Evolution*. She recently retired from teaching middle school science in Miami-Dade County Public Schools after 33 years in the classroom. She is the recipient of several national and local honors, including the NCSE's 2023 Friends of Darwin Award, Samsung's 2014 $150,000 Solve For Tomorrow Contest, and the 2017 winner of the National Association of Biology Teachers Evolution Education Award.

Jonie B. Welland, MA, is a third-year Doctoral Student in School Psychology at the University of Missouri.

Alixandra Wilens, MA, is a Research Assistant for the Yale OCD Research Clinic within the Department of Psychiatry, Yale School of Medicine.

Brian A. Zaboski, PhD, is a Licensed Psychologist and Nationally Ceritfiied School Psychologist, the Director of the Bridgeport Hospital REACH program's Adult Intensive Outpatient Program for OCD and Anxiety, and the Associate Director for Clinical Psychology at the Yale OCD Research Clinic within the Department of Psychiatry, The Yale School of Medicine.

Foreword

Bertha Vazquez

I became familiar with the work of Dr. Stephen Hupp thanks to his articles in *Skeptical Inquirer* magazine. This led me to his books on pseudoscience in pop psychology and child development. His co-editor, Dr. Michael Axelrod, is a professor of psychology at the University of Wisconsin–Eau Claire with years of experience in school psychology. This book is a natural extension of Dr. Hupp's interest in pseudoscience and Dr. Axelrod's search for evidence-based practices in school psychology. They have compiled a team of psychologists questioning many of the practices implemented in school settings.

My first reaction when the editors asked me to write a Foreword for this book was to ask why. Am I qualified? I am not a school psychologist. My last academic foray into the field was as an undergraduate who minored in psychology in the late 1980s. As I read the chapters, however, the reason became clear. As a public school teacher with 33 years of middle school classroom experience, I could see the faces of real children on every page of this book. Every topic came alive. I recalled the children sent home with infant simulation dolls for years. Their science teacher was a big believer in this type of sex education. Countless cheerleaders, musicians, and drama club members have participated in the annual DARE assemblies in our school auditorium. I had to teach the DARE curriculum in my class for years. Furthermore, every year, my students take a statewide assessment that has nothing to do with the subject matter I teach.

Would it surprise the public that instruction does not always drive assessment? When it comes to state exams, it is often the other way around. These one-day assessments can determine a student's academic track for years. The questions raised in this book have daily, real-life consequences for our children.

Ask any K12 teacher to count the hours they have spent in professional development sessions discussing learning styles, the importance of student self-esteem, and other questionable school-related programs, and they will likely say it's too many to count. At best, these are hundreds of hours wasted, which could have been used more effectively. At worst, many of these programs and neuromyths have failed to improve our students' learning or mental health. Many of these programs have sadly directed considerable amounts of money away from evidence-based strategies in a historically low-funded field. Furthermore, several of the therapies discussed in this book can potentially create lasting damage to people. It is agonizing to consider the false hopes given to desperate parents by the now debunked approach called *facilitated communication*. Zero-tolerance programs have inadvertently kept struggling students out of school, putting them even further behind their peers academically.

One phrase in the book struck me: many of these psychological myths are "deeply entrenched in our school culture." This is accurate. So entrenched, in fact, that even those of us primed to question claims made without evidence passively accept them. I joined the Richard Dawkins Foundation for Reason & Science (RDFRS) eight years ago as the director of the Teacher Institute for Evolutionary Science. The RDFRS is now under the umbrella of The Center for Inquiry, an organization specifically created by skeptical thinkers, including Carl Sagan and Isaac Asimov, to promote science and reason and investigate all claims made without evidence. Yet, while I admit to having had suspicions about learning styles for decades, I never asked any presenter to cite the peer-reviewed data. Sadly, it's just not something teachers are typically trained to do. It's not surprising that the authors point out that pseudoscientific practices get minimal attention in graduate school textbooks about school psychology. Not alerting future professionals to possible pseudoscience means that these strategies often make their way into school administrators' and counselors' offices and classrooms. This book should be required reading not just for future school psychologists but for educators as well. As a reader yourself, I encourage you to share the findings chronicled within these pages with your school communities.

Preface

Stephen Hupp

A few days prior to writing this Preface, I accepted a new job as the editor of *Skeptical Inquirer: The Magazine for Science and Reason*. I share this news for two primary reasons. First, I would admittedly love to see an increase in subscriptions by school psychologists – rest assured there will be plenty of discussion about education and psychology in this magazine for years to come. Second, I'd like to acknowledge that a big reason I received the job offer was because of my work on the Investigating Psychology Pseudoscience series. I co-edited the first book – *Investigating Pop Psychology* – with Richard Wisemanand the second book – *Investigating Clinical Psychology* – with Jonathan Stea.

It's okay if you haven't read those first two books before diving into this third book – *Investigating School Psychology* (co-edited with Michael Axelrod). Much like episodes of Black Mirror (or the Twilight Zone), you don't need to experience these books in any particular order. The books in this series have another similarity with Black Mirror: most of the chapters represent some of the darker sides of human nature. That is to say, many people spend a lot of time trying to deceive you with pseudoscientific claims. This book will address several claims related to school psychology that are clearly pseudoscientific. Now it's true that sometimes people making false claims really do believe the claims for themselves, and so we must acknowledge this reality too. Moreover, there are many claims, on the fringe, that might just need more research before a controversy can be fully considered.

We hope this book will be helpful to all school psychologists and to all students of school psychology. Almost every other school psychology book in the world focuses on what school psychologists *should know*. Our book, on the other hand, takes the extremely rare approach of focusing on what school psychologists *should not know*, or at least what school psychologists should be cautious about. That's not to say that everything discussed in this book is *pseudoscience*, per se, but there is plenty of pseudoscience to consider. To a lesser extent, the book also shares evidence-based practices in school psychology to help provide a comparison of what can result from well done research.

Part I of this book introduces science and skepticism by using Chapter 1 to describe some of the cognitive errors and fallacies most relevant to school psychology such as diagnostic overshadowing and pathology bias. Chapter 2 reviews some historical examples of pseudoscience in schools including forced handedness, dunce caps, open classrooms, and the self-esteem movement.

Part II includes three chapters about system-level practices. Chapter 3 examines claims related to zero-tolerance policies, and Chapter 4 describes misconceptions related to suicide prevention. Chapter 5 critically evaluates prevention programs for risky behaviors such as Drug Abuse Resistance Education (DARE), Fatal Vision goggles, abstinence-only sex education, and infant simulator dolls.

Part III focuses on assessment. Chapter 6 tackles questionable claims related to cognitive assessment, and Chapter 7 describes misperceptions about academic assessment. Chapter 8 wraps up the section by doing a deep dive into projective drawing techniques such as the Draw-A-Person, Kinetic Family Drawing, and House-Tree-Person.

Part IV covers classroom instruction and intervention. Chapter 9 describes neuromyths in academic instruction with learning styles as a primary example. Chapter 10 tackles claims related to academic interventions such as kinesiology and vision therapies, and Chapter 11 examines research related to working memory training.

Part V considers topics related to specific populations. Chapter 12 summarizes research on sensory integration, auditory integration, and facilitated communication for children with neurodevelopmental disorders. Chapter 13 examines claims related to behavior problems, and Chapter 14 examines claims related to depression and anxiety.

The Postscript concludes by highlighting practices for youth that have the most research support, so if you ever find yourself getting discouraged then feel free to skip to the end of the book for a little pick-me-up! (Spoiler alert: there are a lot of evidence-based practices in school psychology).

An amazing lineup of experts wrote all of these chapters, and the large majority of them have both an applied background in school psychology as well as a strong grasp of research. We're also delighted to have a Foreword from Bertha Vazquez, a middle school science teacher who became the Director of Education at the Center for Inquiry and editor of the book, *On Teaching Evolution*.

As you read this book, it will help to keep a few additional points in mind adapted from the flagship book in the series – *Investigating Pop Psychology*. That is, knowing the key sources of false beliefs, also called

"The Faker's Dozen," will help you understand why people believe so many dubious claims.

Table: Sources of False Beliefs: The Faker's Dozen

Source of False Beliefs	Definition
Post Hoc Ergo Propter Hoc Reasoning	Believing that one variable caused another variable simply because the first variable occurred before the second variable.
Assuming Causation from Correlation	Believing that one variable caused the other just because they are correlated with each other.
Reasoning by Representativeness	Making a connection between two concepts based on a superficial similarity between them.
Argument from Authority	Arguing that something is true just because an "expert" claimed it to be so (claims made by celebrities are also included in this type of faulty thinking).
False Analogy	Explaining an idea by comparing it to a similar idea while ignoring key unsaid differences.
False Dichotomy	Depicting only two options when there are actually more than two.
Nirvana Fallacy	Assuming that something is completely bad simply because it's not perfect.
Grain of Truth Exaggeration	Making a grand claim based on the fact that only a small aspect of the claim is true.
Appeal to Nature	Arguing that a practice is safer because it's natural.
Appeal to Antiquity	Arguing that a practice is effective simply because it has been used for a long time.
Biased Sample Misperception	Believing we have a full picture of a phenomenon even though we've only been exposed to a specific portion of the phenomenon.
Selective Perception	Perceiving (and recalling) situations that conform to our ideas while failing to notice (or forgetting) situations that are contrary to our ideas.
Confirmation Bias	Seeking out only information that confirms our beliefs while ignoring information that contradicts our beliefs.

Note: This table was adapted from Hupp (2023) which was influenced by several other sources (Hupp & Jewell, 2015; Lilienfeld et al., 2010; Novella et al., 2018; Shermer, 1997).

In addition to those sources, knowing the hallmarks of false claims, also called "The Mucky Seven," can help you be on the lookout for red flags about dubious claims. Recognizing these hallmarks will help you begin with skepticism as you consider both old and new practices in school psychology. Skepticism is the starting point of good science in that scientists actually try to prove themselves wrong, and it's through this process that the best ideas ultimately emerge.

Table: Hallmarks of False Claims: The Mucky Seven

Hallmark of False Claims	Definition
Meaningless Jargon	Incorporating scientific-sounding words that don't have any real connection to the proposed concept. For example, words like "quantum," have real meaning in certain situations, but these words are often used to make a pseudoscientific concept sound more scientific.
Untestable Idea Promotion	Endorsing statements that are not able to be studied through sound research designs. For example, there aren't research study designs that can test many of Freud's concepts.
Anecdote Overreliance	Putting anecdotes ahead of research studies. For example, testimonials are one type of anecdotes that are often used to promote questionable treatments.
Placebo Exploitation	Relying on improvements that occur simply because people know they are getting a treatment. For example, people have the expectation that a treatment will help them get better so they start to feel better once the treatment starts regardless of which treatment is being provided.
Data Manipulation	Using problematic practices related to analyzing and reporting data. For example, when people make dubious claims, they often cherry-pick the data that favors their hypothesis and leave out the rest of the data.
Burden of Proof Shift	Offering a defense by suggesting that it's the skeptics that need to prove them wrong. For example, a psychic might suggest that a skeptic cannot point to research that disproves someone had lived a previous life.
Science Discreditation	Offering a defense by attacking different aspects of science. For example, those making dubious claims often harshly critique the peer-review process.

Note: This table was adapted from Hupp (2023) which was influenced by several other sources (Hupp, 2019; Lilienfeld et al., 2014; Novella et al., 2018; Sagan, 1996).

References

Hupp, S. (2019). *Pseudoscience in child and adolescent psychotherapy: A skeptical field guide.* Cambridge University Press.

Hupp, S., & Jewell, J. (2015). *Great myths of child development.* Wiley.

Hupp, S., & Wiseman, R. (2023). *Investigating pop psychology: Pseudoscience, fringe science, and controversies*. Routledge Press.

Lilienfeld, S. O., In Lynn, S. J., & In Lohr, J. M. (2014). *Science and pseudoscience in clinical psychology*. The Guildford Press.

Lilienfeld, S. O., Lynn, S. J., Ruscio, J., & Beyerstein, B. L. (2010). *50 great myths of popular psychology: Shattering widespread misconceptions about human behavior*. John Wiley & Sons Ltd.

Novella, S., Novella, B., Santa, M. C., Novella, J., & Bernstein, E. (2018). *The skeptics' guide to the universe: How to know what's really real in a world increasingly full of fake*. Grand Central Publishing.

Sagan, C. (1996). *The demon-haunted world: Science as a candle in the dark*. Ballantine Books.

Shermer, M. (1997). *Why people believe weird things*. W.H. Freeman and Co.

Stea, J. N, & Hupp, S. (2023). *Investigating pop psychology: Pseudoscience, fringe science, and controversies*. Routledge Press.

Vazquez, B. (2021). *On teaching evolution*. Keystone Canyon Press.

Acknowledgments

We are grateful to Scott O. Lilienfeld and Steven Jay Lynn for including us as authors in their Great Myths of Psychology book series. Many thanks also to Bertha Vazquez for supporting this project by writing the Foreword, and we are especially thankful to all of the authors who used their expertise to write the engaging chapters to follow.

Many people at Routledge also deserve considerable gratitude. Lucy McClune commissioned the first book in the series and helped expand the project beyond that first book. Danielle Dyal then contracted this book, and Adam Woods helped guide our work throughout much of the journey. Many thanks also to Zoe Thomson for seeing this book through to completion during the final stages of development. We are also indebted to Madeleine Gray for her help with various aspects of this series. Manmohan Negi was a great help as the project manager who organized the final edits. Nupur Bansal was also a superb copyeditor. Many of the strengths of this book are due to all of their combined efforts.

Finally, we would like to thank our colleagues for providing unwavering support and pushing us to think critically about the world in which we live: Drs. April Bleske-Rechek, Melissa Coolong-Chaffin, Mary Beth Tusing (University of Wisconsin-Eau Claire), and Jeremy Jewell (Southern Illinois University Edwardsville).

Part I

Introduction

1 School Psychology, Pseudoscience, and Self-Correction

Michael I. Axelrod

There are a great many concepts and practices in education and psychology that have been largely discredited by science, and a few examples are provided in the book *Investigating Pop Psychology* (Hupp & Wiseman, 2023). No evidence supports Freud's assertion that adult psychopathology is rooted in the child's failure to navigate the psychosexual stages, and critical components of his theory (e.g., Oedipal complex) are generally considered obsolete (Axelrod & Vriesema, 2023). Additionally, the notion that individuals learn better when information is presented in a preferred learning style has serious conceptual and methodological weaknesses (Marshik & Cerbin, 2023). Yet over 350 books and 2,000 academic journal articles on defense mechanisms (a Freudian concept associated with unresolved conflicts occurring during stages of psychosexual development) and psychotherapy were published between 2001 and 2021 (Axelrod & Vriesema, 2023), and an overwhelming majority of educators and the public believe that individual learning styles exist (Macdonald et al., 2017; Newton & Salvi, 2020). While much has been written about how and why (e.g., confirmation bias, illusory correlation, and groupthink) people believe in pseudoscience and fringe science related to psychology, the fact remains that many people, including those in psychology, accept unsupported claims as true.

School psychologists are not immune to misconceptions about psychology or education. A 1997 special issue of *School Psychology Review* focused on exposing several fallacies about students with behavior and learning difficulties (see Berninger, 1997). Topics included the assumed neurobiological etiology of attention-deficit/hyperactivity disorder (ADHD), the use of standardized academic achievement assessments to inform instruction, the view that beginning readers should use context and picture clues when learning to read, and the idea that talking about suicide with children and adolescents is dangerous. More recently, Axelrod et al. (2019) found that practicing school psychologists were generally able to discern facts about child psychology from common myths. However, they also found that more than half of respondents endorsed the following myths as true: "the

DOI: 10.4324/9781003266181-2

Attachment Parenting approach strengthens the mother-infant bond," "most toddlers go through a terrible two's stage," and "a child's drawings provide insight into the subconscious cause of their problems." Hupp et al. (2017) found similar results, as 80% of college students and parents endorsed those five myths as true, suggesting a pervasive belief exists that these ideas have some scientific merits. People, including school psychologists, might be more susceptible to endorsing these five misconceptions as true, as these ideas are often backed by celebrities and experts (e.g., several prominent pediatricians and well-known actors claim attachment parenting supports stronger parent-child relationships) and promoted via word of mouth (e.g., consider the familiar phrase "terrible twos"). The study also found that acceptance of these myths did not differ across education levels (i.e., Educational Specialist vs. Doctorate) or years of experience suggesting education and experience might not protect school psychologists from believing certain myths.

Possibly most noteworthy from the Axelrod et al. (2019) study was that more than half of school psychologists endorsed the idea that a child's drawing could offer insights into the subconscious causes of problems. This myth originates from the idea that children's drawings possess features helpful in recognizing psychological problems and diagnosing psychological disorders. School psychology scholars have criticized evaluation practices involving children's drawings, principally because of their poor psychometric qualities, poor incremental and predictive validity, and questionable practicality when planning interventions (Miller, 2010; Motta et al., 1993). Yet, school psychologists continue to use children's drawings to form hypotheses about problems and make decisions about children (see Hojnoski et al., 2006; Shapiro & Heick, 2004). Axelrod et al. (2019) also found that years of experience were unrelated to the propensity to believe children's drawings could offer insights into the subconscious causes of problems. Said differently, school psychologists trained within the last decade were not less likely to believe this myth when compared to school psychologists trained 20 or more years ago. School psychology graduate programs are urged to teach about assessment instruments with strong psychometric properties, especially when making decisions about students. In addition, professional development promoted regionally and nationally often addresses the reliable and valid assessment of behavior and social/emotional functioning. Yet, research described above suggests school psychologists may be engaging in practices that are inconsistent with science. For more about projective drawings, see Chapter 8 of this book.

Scholars have presented evidence of a research-practice gap in school psychology (e.g., Forman et al., 2009; Lilienfeld et al., 2012). While this gap may represent a knowledge gap, misconceptions about certain ideas in school psychology (and education and child development more broadly) might also play a role. Critical thinking, including the skill of discerning fact from fiction, in school psychology is especially important. Lilienfeld et al. (2012) highlighted several examples where school psychologists' use of unsupported practices might cause harm (e.g., misdiagnosis of learning disabilities based on interpretations of intelligence test subtest profiles, the opportunity costs associated with implementation of ineffective suicide prevention programs). Fortunately, understanding how people come to believe unsupported claims or engage in pseudoscientific practices might offer a framework for closing the research-practice gap that exists in school psychology.

Cognitive Errors and Fallacies Relevant to School Psychology

There are many reasons school psychologists might believe in myths related to psychology or engage in practices considered pseudoscientific or based on fringe science. Moreover, there are many controversies in the fields of school psychology and, more broadly, education that complicate the practice landscape. Engaging in critical and scientific thinking about these topics and practices might shield school psychologists from the hazards of pseudoscience, fringe science, and controversy. Scholars have pointed to common errors in thinking as sources of false beliefs. As a starting point for considering many claims made in psychology, Hupp (2023) presents the "Faker's Dozen," 13 types of cognitive errors inspired by the "sources of psychological myths" from Lilienfeld et al. (2010).

Lilienfeld et al. (2012) offered additional cognitive errors and biases relevant to school psychologists. These cognitive errors can impact practice including decision-making and the types and quality of services delivered by professionals. Featherston et al. (2020) conducted a review of existing research to explore whether decisions (e.g., assessment, diagnostic, and treatment) made by allied health professionals, including psychologists, were shaped by cognitive, affective, or other biases (e.g., stereotyping bias, confirmation bias). The reviewed studies used hypothetical scenarios to investigate how bias influenced professionals' decision-making. The researchers found that 77% of the 149 reviewed studies reported outcomes indicating the existence of bias in decision outcomes. School psychologists may be most susceptible to cognitive errors when engaging in the special education referral process to make special education eligibility decisions (Watkins, 2009).

The remainder of this section highlights three common cognitive errors relevant to school psychology practice and two related fallacies that might perpetuate pseudoscience and fringe science.

Diagnostic Overshadowing

Imagine working with a high school student with a diagnosis of ADHD. Inattention and poor work completion are the primary presenting problems. Observing the student, you notice they are frequently off-task and inattentive. You conclude that inattention and poor work completion are linked to the student's previously diagnosed ADHD. This tendency of interpreting presenting problems based on previous diagnoses (i.e., ADHD) and failing to investigate other potential causes (e.g., the student's inattention is a function of frequent and intense worry about school performance) is called diagnostic overshadowing.

Reiss et al. (1982) initially used the term diagnostic overshadowing to describe how healthcare professionals might incorrectly attribute symptoms (e.g., worry, sadness, and attention problems) to intellectual disability (ID) rather than comorbid psychiatric disorders (e.g., generalized anxiety disorder, major depressive disorder, and ADHD). The concept has since been broadened to suggest how a primary diagnosis may reduce the importance of a secondary diagnosis. For example, the presence of autism spectrum disorder (ASD) may result in a clinician regarding symptoms of anxiety as features of ASD and, thus, overlooking a diagnosis of anxiety and interventions specific to anxiety. In their review of existing research, Jopp and Keys (2001) found that diagnostic overshadowing "is a robust clinical phenomenon that is relatively unaffected by a wide variety of variables" (p. 431) and likely happening in practice.

Goldsmith and Schloss (1986) studied diagnostic overshadowing among school psychologists working with students with hearing impairments. After reviewing case descriptions of students with hearing impairments, school psychologists were more likely to use terms like *tense* and *depressed* to describe presenting problems, while those reviewing case descriptions involving students without hearing impairments or other disabilities applied diagnostic labels such as *learning disability* and *behavioral disorder*. Perhaps more importantly, school psychologists in the hearing impairment condition were more likely to recommend nonspecific interventions (e.g., academic support, home involvement), whereas those in the nondisability condition were more likely to recommend specific interventions targeting learning and behavior. More recently, Sullivan et al. (2019) investigated school psychologists' special education eligibility decision-making related to emotional disability, ID, and ASD. The researchers found that, across eligibility categories, school psychologists made decisions inconsistent with eligibility criteria, ignoring important data critical to each category in favor of more salient features. For example, school psychologists were far more likely to render a diagnosis of ID only when a cognitive impairment was present versus not present despite clear indications the student presented with behaviors consistent with ASD. Sullivan et al. (2019) described this phenomenon as overshadowing and suggested it might explain why ASD prevalence in special education is lower than that reported across clinical settings.

Diagnostic overshadowing can affect school psychologists' clinical decision-making in three primary provinces – severity of symptoms, special education category or diagnosis, and treatment. Scholars agree that differential and dual diagnoses are complicated features of psychological disorders, and comorbidity is the rule not the exception in child and adolescent psychopathology. Yet, accurately evaluating symptom severity by direct measures, minimizing false positives through reliable and valid assessment, and designing interventions to address specific behaviors rather than broad diagnostic categories seem prudent ways of diminishing diagnostic overshadowing's impact.

Unpacking Failure

When evaluating students referred for reading problems, especially older students, school psychologists often rely exclusively on screening and standardized assessment data when making decisions. However, students struggling to read often have underlying language challenges (e.g., poor phonological awareness). That is, a school psychologist's failure to elicit all relevant information, including language ability, may result in noteworthy possibilities being overlooked. This example illustrates unpacking failure, a common cognitive error involving the failure to obtain all relevant information when conceptualizing a problem or establishing a diagnosis. The unpacking principle states "that a more detailed description of an implicit hypothesis generally increases its judged probability" (Watkins et al., 2018, p. 1199). In practice, the principle implies that more information about a problem enhances clinical reasoning and decision-making and that failing to do so results in important possibilities being discounted or missed. This "unpacking" of information facilitates a clinician's decision-making strategy.

Unpacking failure is widespread in practice settings. Croskerry and Campbell (2021) found the failure of physicians to gather all relevant assessment data to be one of the more frequent emergency department diagnostic mistakes – more frequent than even knowledge deficits (e.g., not being aware of certain diagnostic criteria common to a particular disease). In school psychology, where large amounts of data are available and multiple informants are used to assess students, unpacking failure can be commonplace. Allen and Hanchon (2013) demonstrated this by studying the assessment practices of school psychologists when evaluating students referred for emotional disturbance. The researchers found that just over one-quarter of participants included two or fewer critical assessment components (i.e., parent interview, teacher interview, student interview, observation, and behavior rating scales), rather than taking a multimethod approach. In a separate study, Hanchon and Allen (2013) found that school psychologists rarely moved beyond behavior rating scales when making decisions about students referred for special education eligibility under the emotional disturbance category. These researchers suggested that moving school psychology forward when considering the identification of students with emotional disturbance must involve, among other things, attending to and protecting against cognitive errors like unpacking failure.

There are several hypotheses as to why unpacking failure might occur so frequently. First, school psychologists may gather just enough information to confirm eligibility for special education services. Consequences of this practice might include misidentification of a student's disability category and inadequate and/or insufficient data to inform intervention planning. Second, too much information may disable the decision-making process. School psychologists may find multiple sources of conflicting data difficult to interpret leading to feelings of being stuck. Finally, weak federal and state definitions (e.g., social maladjustment and emotional disturbance) and ambiguous procedural guidelines (e.g., response to intervention) might influence a school psychologist's conceptualization of what data are needed to make decisions and place limits on what information a school psychologist finds helpful.

Pathology Bias

Sigmund Freud suggested that psychological disorders were rooted in a child's experiences navigating psychosexual stages of development (e.g., oral, anal, and phallic). His theory implied that children's experiences with toilet training would profoundly affect personality and that delays in successfully achieving continence represented underlying emotional disturbances (Axelrod & Vriesema, 2023). Although research demonstrates that children late to complete toilet training are no different psychologically than their toilet-trained peers (Axelrod et al., 2021), the idea that delays in toilet training are associated with psychological problems appears to be a widely held belief (Fruit et al., 2019). This example represents a frequent cognitive bias, the pathology bias, or the tendency to pathologize or overinterpret relatively common problems.

Friman and Blum (2002) provided several other examples of childhood problems that often reflect what they termed "clinical normality" and not psychopathology including chronic hair pulling, thumb sucking, and childhood fears. These common childhood problems are represented on a continuum of normality and research on the psychopathology of these problems rarely finds significant group differences (i.e., groups of children with and without the presenting problem) except for a small subgroup of extreme cases. These extreme cases, however, become sources for psychology's conceptualization of these childhood problems. Extreme cases are more likely to be included as data in published research (known as Berkson's bias or a selection bias where a sample is taken from a subgroup and not the general population) and used as teaching examples (known as the textbook bias) where extreme cases might provide students with more valuable learning experiences than everyday cases. Because of these biases, practitioners orient their assessment, diagnostic, and treatment practices toward the extreme cases rather than attempting to first understand the presenting problems as a slight variation of normal.

The pathology bias has been a long-time fixture in psychology and psychiatry (e.g., classifying homosexuality as a disorder, recommending treatment for people experiencing a normal reaction to grief) and regarding normal life experiences as pathological influences how our culture responds to them. For school psychologists, this bias may be represented in evaluation practices (e.g., assessment instruments may be biased toward finding pathology) and the process for determining eligibility for special education services (e.g., meeting criteria for an educational disability is the initial step to receiving services; Weist, 2003). For example, research has found that projective personality assessments (e.g., Rorschach Inkblots, Thematic Apperception Test) overpathologize what is generally considered normal behavior (see Hines, 2023) and certain procedures for identifying specific learning disabilities (SLDs), such as interpreting profiles of strengths and weaknesses in cognitive skills, have a tendency to overidentify students (Cottrell & Barrett, 2016).

Argumentum ad Antiquitatem and ad Populum Fallacies

The reauthorization of Individuals with Disabilities Education Act (IDEA) in 2004 brought significant changes to the procedure in which SLDs are identified. The IQ/Achievement Discrepancy model (i.e., determining whether SLDs are present based on whether a substantial difference exists between scores on a cognitive and academic achievement assessment) was discontinued due to the lack of empirical evidence supporting its validity in favor of a framework featuring response to scientifically based instruction and intervention. Despite IDEA allowing school districts to stop mandating cognitive assessment for SLD, assessment practices among school psychologists have hardly changed as a result (Benson et al., 2019). The appeal to tradition or *argumentum ad antiquitatem* (argument for antiquity) might help explain why school psychologists continue to administer cognitive assessments when addressing referral concerns related to an SLD. This common logic fallacy occurs when a claim is said to be true only because it has been around for a while. The tendency to believe a practice is effective or valid because of its popularity (i.e., the *ad populum fallacy* or appeal to people) might also account for school psychologists' enduring use of cognitive assessments. There are many other instances in education and, more specifically, school psychology where the attractiveness of tradition and popularity might explain pseudoscientific practices and beliefs. For example, the continued use of projective tests (e.g., Rorschach Inkblots, Thematic Apperception Test, children's drawings), which lack adequate reliability and validity to be of clinical utility, likely has something to do with tradition and popularity (Hines, 2023). Many pseudoscientific practices in education are rooted in these fallacies. Teaching students based on their individual learning styles (or whether they are right- or left-brained) and whole-language approaches to reading instruction remain popular features of the educational landscape despite a lack of evidence for their support.

A more thorough discussion of a common practice might further illustrate how appeals to tradition and popularity might perpetuate unsupported practices in school psychology. Cognitive profile analysis involves constructing inferences about students' strengths and weaknesses based on a cognitive assessment's individual subtest patterned score variation. While the precise origin of this interpretive approach is largely unknown, documented procedures using cognitive profile analysis have been recognized in clinical and school psychology since before World War II. Studies conducted in the 1990s questioned the practice's psychometric and theoretical foundation leading scholars to conclude cognitive profile analysis lacked sufficient scientific evidence and clinical utility (see McGill et al., 2018 for a more thorough discussion). Yet, the practice remains popular with school psychologists. A survey of school psychologists around 2000 indicated that almost 90% regularly used profile analysis when interpreting cognitive assessments (Pfeiffer et al., 2000). Almost 20 years later, national surveys of assessment practices among school psychologists suggest that approximately half of respondents engage in profile analysis (McGill et al., 2018). These more recent findings should be surprising. While there has been a notable decline in the use of cognitive profile analysis, many school psychologists continue engaging in the practice despite the evidence. Perhaps school psychologists' belief that profile analysis has scientific merit is based, in part, on history and popularity. A further examination of profile analysis' acceptance in school psychology points to graduate training and instructional materials as being partially responsible for perpetuating the tradition and widespread acceptance of this interpretive approach. As recently as five years ago, many instructors teaching cognitive assessment courses still emphasized various versions of profile analysis (Lockwood & Farmer, 2020). Moreover, commonly used instructional materials (e.g., textbooks, chapters, and assessment manuals) within school psychology – and that have become teaching aids in those cognitive assessment courses – often provide interpretive recommendations consistent with profile analysis (Farmer et al., 2021). To summarize, the tendency to believe something is valid because it has been around for a while or is popular could explain why some school psychologists believe cognitive profile analysis is a scientifically sound practice.

Summary and Conclusions

This chapter presented evidence that school psychology is not invulnerable to practices based on pseudoscience or fringe science. In fact, there are a great deal of practices occurring in school psychology, and education more broadly, that have little or no scientific support. Perhaps more alarming is many of these practices continue despite the accumulation of data, over decades in some cases, refuting their scientific and applied value. This chapter also provided examples from school psychology where cognitive errors and fallacies help explain how practices based on nonsense might persist. These errors in thinking represent just a few of the many widespread biases, heuristics, and misconceptions derailing school psychologists from engaging in evidence-based practices.

Ioannidis (2012) wrote that self-correction is a fundamental characteristic of any scientific discipline and that scientific credibility results from efficient and unbiased replication that exists as a mechanism of self-correction. Yet, school psychology and other related applied fields (e.g., clinical psychology, educational psychology), which claim to be grounded in science, seem to lack the capacity to properly self-correct. The continued use of projective drawings and cognitive profile analysis, despite questionable theoretical and scientific foundations, offers some evidence that school psychology has failed to self-correct, at least regarding these two practices. Consequences of this failure to self-correct are significant. Most notably, practices and ideas based on pseudoscience or fringe science are harmful to children and families, as many of the topics in this book highlight.

There are several ways school psychologists can protect themselves from believing in pseudoscience and engaging in dubious practices. Approaching ideas with a critical (or sometimes skeptical) eye, sharpening critical thinking skills, being aware of our tendency toward cognitive errors and the overreliance on heuristics (i.e., mental shortcuts), accepting uncertainty in our knowledge base, and recognizing the limits of science are some habits that might promote evidence-based practices and close the science-practice gap afflicting school psychology and education. This book is an expedition into pseudoscience, fringe science, and the many controversies existing in school psychology. It attempts to investigate common topics relevant to school psychology practice, stimulate critical thinking, and be a catalyst for much-needed self-correction.

References

Allen, R. A., & Hanchon, T. A. (2013). What can we learn from school-based emotional disturbance assessment practices? Implications for practice and preparation in school psychology. *Psychology in the Schools, 50*, 290–299.

Axelrod, M. I., Hoffman, C., Latimer, J., & Weber, A. (2019). Fact or fiction: School psychologists' beliefs about myths in psychology. *The WSPA Sentinel, 19*, 18–22.

Axelrod, M. I., Larsen, R. J., Jorgensen, K., & Stratman, B. (2021). Psychological differences between toilet trained and non-toilet trained 4-year-old children. *Journal for Specialists in Pediatric Nursing, 26*, e12319.

Axelrod, M. I., & Vriesema, C. C. (2023). Psychosexual stages and development. In S. Hupp & R. Wiseman (Eds.), *Investigating pop psychology: Pseudoscience, fringe science, and controversies* (pp. 75–85). Routledge.

Benson, N. F., Floyd, R. G., Kranzler, J. H., Eckert, T. L., Fefer, S. A., & Morgan, G. B. (2019). Test use and assessment practices of school psychologists in the United States: Findings from the 2017 national survey. *Journal of School Psychology, 72*, 29–48.

Berninger, V. W. (1997). Introduction to interventions for students with learning and behavior problems: Myths and realities. *School Psychology Review, 26*, 326–332.

Cottrell, J. M., & Barrett, C. A. (2016). Defining the undefinable: Operationalization of methods to identify specific learning disabilities among practicing school psychologists. *Psychology in the Schools, 53*, 143–157.

Croskerry, P., & Campbell, S. G. (2021). A cognitive autopsy approach towards explaining diagnostic failure. *Cureus, 13*(8), e17041.

Farmer, R. L., McGill, R. J., Dombrowski, S. C., & Canivez, G. L. (2021). Why questionable assessment practices remain popular in school psychology: Instructional materials as pedagogical vehicles. *Canadian Journal of School Psychology, 36*, 98–114.

Featherston, R., Downie, L. E., Vogel, A. P., & Galvin, K. L. (2020). Decision making biases in the allied health professions: A systematic scoping review. *PLoS ONE, 15*(10), e0240716.

Forman, S. G., Fagley, N.S., Steiner, D. D., & Schneider, K. (2009). Teaching evidence-based interventions: Perceptions of influences on use in professional practice in school psychology. *Training and Education in Professional Psychology, 3*, 226–232.

Friman, P. C., & Blum, N. (2002). Primary care behavioral pediatrics. In M. Hersen & W. Sledge (Eds.), *Encyclopedia of psychotherapy, Vol 2* (pp. 379–399). Academic Press.

Fruit, N. A., Jorgensen, K. J., Helwig, E. C., George, K. J., Schmidt, C. K., & Axelrod, M. I. (2019, August). Fact or fiction: Pre-professionals' beliefs about child psychology myths. Presentation at the Annual Convention of the American Psychological Association, Chicago, IL.

Goldsmith, L., & Schloss, P.J. (1986). Diagnostic overshadowing among school psychologists working with hearing-impaired learners. *American Annals of the Deaf, 131,* 288–293.

Hanchon, T. A., & Allen, R. A. (2013). Identifying students with emotional disturbance: School psychologists' practices and perceptions. *Psychology in the Schools, 50,* 193–208.

Hines, T. (2023). Projective tests and personality. In S. Hupp & R. Wiseman (Eds.), *Investigating pop psychology: Pseudoscience, fringe science, and controversies* (pp. 121–129). Routledge.

Hojnoski, R. L., Morrison, R., Brown, M., & Matthews, W. (2006). Projective test use among school psychologists: A survey and critique. *Journal of Psychoeducational Assessment, 24,* 145–159.

Hupp, S. (2023). Examining claims in pop psychology. In S. Hupp & R. Wiseman (Eds.), *Investigating pop psychology: Pseudoscience, fringe science, and controversies* (pp. 1–8). Routledge.

Hupp, S., Stary, A., & Jewell, J. (2017). Science vs. silliness for parents: Debunking the myths of child psychology. *Skeptical Inquirer, 41(1),* 44–47.

Hupp, S., & Wiseman, R. (2023). *Investigating pop psychology: Pseudoscience, fringe science, and controversies.* Routledge.

Ioannidis, J. P. A. (2012). Why science is not necessarily self-correcting. *Perspectives on Psychological Science, 7,* 645–654.

Jopp, D. A., & Keys, C. B. (2001). Diagnostic overshadowing reviewed and reconsidered. *American Journal on Mental Retardation, 106,* 146–433.

Lilienfeld, S. O., Ammirati, R., & David, M. (2012). Distinguishing science from pseudoscience in school psychology: Science and scientific thinking as safeguards against human error. *Journal of School Psychology, 50,* 7–36.

Lilienfeld, S. O., Lynn, S. J., Ruscio, J., & Beyerstein, B. L. (2010). *50 great myths of popular psychology: Shattering widespread misconceptions about human behavior.* Wiley.

Lockwood, A. B., & Farmer, R. L. (2020). The cognitive assessment course: Two decades later. *Psychology in the Schools, 57,* 265–283.

Macdonald, K., Germine, L., Anderson, A., Christodoulou, J., & McGrath, L. M. (2017). Dispelling the myth: Training in education or neuroscience decreases but does not eliminate beliefs in neuromyths. *Frontiers in Psychology, 8,* 1314.

Marshik, T., & Cerbin, W. (2023). Learning styles and cognition. In S. Hupp & R. Wiseman (Eds.), *Investigating pop psychology: Pseudoscience, fringe science, and controversies* (pp. 56–65). Routledge.

McGill, R. J., Dombrowski, S. C., & Canivez, G. L. (2018). Cognitive profile analysis in school psychology: History, issues, and continued concerns. *Journal of School Psychology, 71,* 108–121.

Miller, D. N. (2010). Assessing internalizing problems and well-being. In G. G. Peacock, R. A. Ervin, E. J. Daly, & K. W. Merrell (Eds.), *Practical handbook of school psychology: Effective practices for the 21st century* (pp. 175–191). Guilford.

Motta, R. W., Little, S. G., & Tobin, M. I. (1993). The use and abuse of human figure drawings. *School Psychology Quarterly, 8*, 162–169.

Newton, P. M., & Salvi, A. (2020). How common is belief in the learning styles neuromyth, and does it matter? A pragmatic systematic review. *Frontiers in Education, 5*, 602451.

Pfeiffer, S. I., Reddy, L. A., Kletzel, J. E., Schmeizer, E. R., & Boyer, L. M. (2000). The practitioner's view of IQ testing and profile analysis. *School Psychology Quarterly, 15*, 376–385.

Reiss, S., Levitan, G., & Szyszko, J. (1982). Emotional disturbance and mental retardation: Diagnostic overshadowing. *American Journal of Mental Deficiency, 86*, 567–574.

Shapiro, E. S., & Heick, P. F. (2004). School psychologist assessment practices in the evaluation of students referred for social/behavioral/emotional problems. *Psychology in the Schools, 41*, 551–561.

Sullivan, A. L., Sadeh, S., & Houri, A.K. (2019). Are school psychologists' special education eligibility decisions reliable and unbiased? A multi-study experimental investigation. *Journal of School Psychology, 77*, 90–109.

Watkins, M. W. (2009). Errors in diagnostic decision making and clinical judgment. In T. B. Gutkin & C. R. Reynolds (Eds.), *Handbook of school psychology* (4th ed.) (pp. 210–229). Wiley.

Watkins, S., Gaffo, A. L., Clark, A. V., & Steinhilber, S. (2018). An exercise in clinical reasoning: Do you unpack? *Journal of General Internal Medicine, 33*, 1196–1200.

Weist, M. D. (2003). Challenges and opportunities in moving toward a public health approach in school mental health. *Journal of School Psychology, 41*, 77–82.

2 Historical Pseudoscience in Schools

Scott Bellini, Parker S. Beckman, and Hanna S. Lim

The history of education has been littered with popular pseudoscience practices that were eventually discarded into the dustbin of ineffectual practices. These pseudoscience practices were once widely accepted and implemented in schools but have since been discredited by empirical evidence and replaced by more effective evidence-based interventions (or in some cases, with other pseudoscience practices). Like all pseudoscience practices, these strategies, and their associated educational "movements," were based on ideas that seemed reasonable at the time, and often leveraged the zeitgeist of popular culture. All of these strategies lacked rigorous research support and empirical validation but were often presented as science, or "research-based" by advocates who misinterpreted, misrepresented, or exploited the available research on the practice.

In this chapter, we will explore four examples of historical pseudoscience practices in school psychology. First, forced handedness refers to the practice of forcing left-handed students to use their right hand when engaged in various school tasks, such as writing. Second, the use of dunce caps was a prominent disciplinary strategy that has been widely captured in popular culture. Third, the self-esteem movement was a widely accepted movement that began in the 1960s and permeated much of popular culture and education for the last three decades of the 20th century. Finally, the open classroom concept came into prominence in the 1970s, and quite literally changed the architectural landscape of schools in America.

Examining the Claims

Forced Handedness

Handedness, or the tendency to be either left- or right-handed (or both), is an important factor in a child's education and development. Though the exact neurobiological structures and processes involved in hand preference remain somewhat unclear, there does appear to be neurobiological basis

DOI: 10.4324/9781003266181-3

for right- and left-handedness (Sha et al., 2021). Hand preference can play a significant role in how a student engages in educational tasks and how they use various learning tools and devices. As such, understanding and accommodating for differences in handedness is an effective way to promote educational success and is something done routinely in schools today. However, well into the 20th century in America and other Western cultures (and still done today in some cultures), many left-handed children were forced to use their right hands in school due to misguided cultural and societal beliefs toward left-handedness (Alhassan, 2017; McManus, 2019).

There are so many recent examples of successful and high-achieving left-handers in American society (e.g., Oprah Winfrey, Bill Gates, Ruth Bader Ginsburg, and Presidents Ford, Reagan, Bush, Obama, and Clinton) that it seems absurd to think that it was once viewed as aberrant. Throughout history, left-handedness has been claimed to be abnormal and deviant in many cultures, leading to the mistreatment and discrimination of left-handed individuals (Alhassan, 2017). For many centuries, it was widely believed that left-handedness was a sign of moral fragility or depravity. In fact, left-handedness was quite literally associated with being sinister, as the Latin translation of the word "sinister" is "on the left-side." In ancient Greece, left-handedness was associated with deceit and wickedness, leading to discrimination and persecution against left-handed individuals. Similarly, in medieval Europe, left-handedness was considered unholy, and associated with the devil, which forced left-handed individuals to hide their handedness for fear of being seen as witches or perhaps practitioners of the dark arts. Though to a lesser extent, these cultural beliefs were perpetuated throughout much of the 20th century as left-handedness was thought to be associated with multiple mental health and learning difficulties (McManus, 2019; Porac, 2016). Even today, the relics of this bias toward left-handedness persist in idioms such as "a left-handed compliment" which generally means "to give a disguised insult."

As a result of these misconceptions, the pseudoscience practice of forcing left-handed students to become right-handed was common in schools in Europe and America in the 19th and 20th centuries. In schools, left-handed students were commonly forced to work with their right hands to "normalize" or hide their handedness. In fact, both President Ford and President Reagan were left-handers who were forced to convert to right-handers by teachers and parents. The claim that prompted this practice was that it would hide their left-handedness and allow them to better fit into a right-hand dominant society where the behavior setting is often designed specifically for right-handed inhabitants. For instance, learning and occupational implements, such as scissors, desk, computer mouse, and various power tools, are intended exclusively for right-handed use.

In addition, western writing is taught from a right-to-left motion which can be quite difficult for left-handed students to learn and execute.

Though the exact frequency of the practice is unknown, these beliefs, and the explicit efforts to "convert" left-handed students were so common that it may have had an impact on the number of left-handers in the total population ... or at least the number of people identifying as left-handed. For instance, only 2% of the population identified as left-handed at the beginning of the 20th century. However, as attitudes toward left-handedness began to shift, and as researchers began to determine that forced handedness was not only unnecessary, but also potentially harmful (McManus, 2019; Terman, 1914), treatment of left-handers slowly began to change throughout the 20th century. Not surprisingly, and perhaps consequently, the rate of left-handers in the population increased steadily during the last century, up to 5% in the 1950s, and eventually to the current rate of approximately 10% (Porac, 2016).

Ironically, the pseudoscience practice of forcing left-handed children to use their right hand may have been derailed by another line of pseudo-science, namely, the erroneous and flawed research that indicated that forcing left-handed children to use the right hand would cause myriad learning difficulties and neurological impairment, including schizophrenia, stuttering, and dyslexia. In fact, this notion was promoted by prominent psychologist, Lewis Terman, who claimed in his widely popular book *The Hygiene of School Children,* that up to a half of all stuttering in school-aged children was a result of forcing left-handed children to become right-handers (1914). This belief was perpetuated by the biographies of natural left-handers, King George VI (as depicted in the movie "The Kings Speech") and Harry S. Truman, which recount tales of how both men developed stuttering or stammering as a result of being forced to convert to right-handers. These claims were echoed by other prominent psychologists of the era who theorized that forcing a left-handed student to become right-handed created an unnatural symmetry of the brain that led to stuttering (McManus, 2019). This view has not been corroborated by subsequent research, much of which has indicated that the practice of forced handedness, although unnecessary, did not lead to lasting harm in most individuals forced to convert (Porac, 2016). Interestingly though, recent research examining the brains of former left-handers forced to convert to right-handers using functional MRI technology has indicated that forcing left-handed children to use their right hand does apparently impact and change various neurobiological structures (Kloppel et al., 2010). However, it's still not clear whether this neurological change is ultimately harmful or beneficial to the individual. In fact, in some cases, forced conversion may have slightly enhanced motor skill functioning by promoting ambidextrous use of hands. However, considering that the practice undoubtedly led to needless stress; conflict between parent, teacher, and student; and behavioral issues – not to mention ruined the Hall of Fame pitching careers of an untold number of natural southpaws – it is a practice that certainly deserves its current place in the rubbish bin of discarded pseudoscience practices.

Dunce Caps

Perhaps no other historical pseudoscience practice in education left a bigger stain on the field than the use of dunce caps. Dunce caps, which were typically used as a disciplinary strategy, were tall conical hats with the word "dunce" or a large "D" written on them. Students were forced to wear these caps if they were deemed to be disruptive or not performing well academically. In addition to wearing a dunce cap, the student was put on "display" in the corner of the room, which meant being excluded from taking part in educational and social activities with classmates.

The practice of using dunce caps in a pejorative sense dates back to the Renaissance era (Weaver, 2012). Interestingly, dunce caps were once worn as a symbol of wisdom, by erudite followers of John Duns Scotus, who was a highly influential philosopher and theologian of the Middle Ages. Duns Scotus believed that the pointed hats would somehow funnel knowledge from the world into his follower's minds. The subsequent Renaissance era was a time of immense cultural, artistic, political, and philosophical change, and with it came a rejection and repudiation of ideas and symbols of the Middle Ages. As such, the dunce cap became a derogatory symbol of Duns Scotus and his followers and subsequently became an established ritual of humiliation in schools throughout England.

Public humiliation and "badge of shame" techniques (think, "The Scarlet Letter") were fully entrenched in society through much of the 19th century (Stearns & Stearns, 2017). Shame-based punishments were routinely doled out in the court system, and not surprisingly, schools mirrored this cultural attitude in their disciplinary practices of students. In fact, "best practices" for corporal punishment of children at the time involved the delivery of physical punishment in the presence of other children. The use of dunce caps fit nicely into this cultural paradigm of public humiliation, and it was a common practice in schools throughout Europe and America from the 16th century until the mid-20th century (Stearns & Stearns, 2017).

Though it is impossible to determine with any precision just how frequently dunce caps were used in American schools, their use certainly left an indelible impression on the consciousness of the American Public. The dunce cap first appeared in literature courtesy of Charles Dickens in his book "The Old Curiosity Shop" in 1840 and was depicted in numerous education texts in the 1800s (Weaver, 2012). Today, the dunce cap remains an iconic symbol of public humiliation in educational settings and society at large. Throughout the 20th century and up to the present time, the use of dunce caps, or references to wearing one, and its association with "dumb" behavior, has been ubiquitously depicted in popular culture, including literature, cartoons, comic strips, movies, and popular television shows, such as *Looney Tunes, Little Rascals, Calvin & Hobbs, Dennis the Menace, Silicon Valley,* and *The Simpsons.*

The rationale behind the educational use of the dunce cap, its real teeth if you will, was that it would shame and humiliate the student into improved classroom behavior and academic performance. And as a form of humiliation, it provided the perfect exemplar of the triangle of humiliation offered by Klein (1991) which includes a public act of humiliation, a target (or victim), and the presence of an audience (or witness). From a behavioral perspective, the dunce cap was used primarily as a punisher for problem behavior. It also served as means to motivate students to do their work, and thus, avoid having to wear the dunce cap. Although no research exists on the use of dunce caps specifically, subsequent research studies have demonstrated that public shaming and humiliation may have an immediate impact on problem behaviors but long-lasting negative effects on a student's mental health, self-esteem, and their attitudes about school in general (Stearns & Stearns, 2017). As attitudes toward public humiliation and shame-based techniques shifted in America during the 20th century, the use of dunce caps decreased and ultimately disappeared from schools and was replaced with more positive forms of discipline such as those advocated by the positive behavior support movement. That said, old habits die hard, and the vestiges of dunce caps and public humiliation lived for many years in practices such as writing children's name on the board and making children sit outside the classroom as punishment of problem behaviors (Stearns & Stearns, 2017).

The use of the dunce cap as a form of punishment and public humiliation in educational settings has virtually vanished in practice and is universally recognized as both absurd and dehumanizing. However, the symbol remains in people's minds as an evocative reminder of the practice of public shaming in schools, and unfortunately, public shaming of students as a disciplinary strategy has persisted in other forms to this present day. Despite the controversy surrounding their use, the historical use of dunce caps provides valuable insight into the evolution of societal norms and their influence on educational practices, and of the changing perspectives on discipline, humiliation, and dignity in our society.

The Self-Esteem Movement

The self-esteem movement was a burgeoning pop psychology phenomenon in the 1970s and consequently, became a popular pseudoscience approach in education throughout the remainder of the 20th century. Self-esteem, which is generally defined as one's views or beliefs about self, or their self-worth, is thought to be an important factor in a person's overall psychological development and well-being. The term "self-esteem" was first introduced as a psychological construct in the 1890s by noted psychologist William James, but it wasn't until the late 1960s and 1970s that it became prevalent in popular culture when American psychologist Nathaniel Branden published his 1969 book *The Psychology of Self-Esteem*. The book provided an alternative, and a complete rebuke, to two prominent conceptual frameworks in psychology at the time, psychoanalysis and behaviorism. Branden framed self-esteem as an important concept for understanding and addressing psychological and emotional issues, noting the importance of "self-acceptance," "self-responsibility," and "believing in oneself" as components of a healthy self-concept (Branden, 2001). By the end of the 20th century, the self-esteem movement had permeated popular culture and helped ignite a multibillion-dollar cottage industry for various authors and motivational speakers who flooded American homes, businesses, and ultimately, schools, with books, workbooks, and educational seminars designed to boost the collective self-esteem of American citizens (Singal, 2017).

Emboldened by a growing body of correlational research from the 1970s and 1980s which highlighted associations between self-esteem and numerous other outcomes, proponents of the movement claimed, quite adamantly, that enhancing students' self-esteem would lead to improved academic, social, emotional, behavioral, and occupational performance (Branden, 1984; Mecca et al., 1989). The movement reached its full height in the state of California in the 1980s when then Governor George Deukmejian established a well-publicized (and well-funded) task force on self-esteem (Baumeister et al., 2005). One prominent state representative, who was the most vocal champion of the movement and member of the task force, John Vasconcellos, hypothesized that improving self-esteem in California school children would help to balance the state budget as it was believed that people with high self-regard make more money, and thus pay more in taxes. The task force developed a working paper titled, *The Social Importance of Self-Esteem* (Mecca et al., 1989), that concluded that raising self-esteem could lead to improved school achievement, and a reduction in crime, teen pregnancy, and drug abuse. However, the task force, and the movement in general, was based on a misunderstanding of the construct of self-esteem, and like other pseudoscience approaches, an apparent inability to discern between correlation and causation. While the self-esteem movement has faded in prominence, a review of the research suggests that it may have done more harm than good (Baumeister et al., 2005).

Several studies over the years (Baumeister et al., 2003; Diener & Diener, 1995; Hansford & Hattie, 1982; Pottebaum et al., 1986) have shown significant correlations between self-esteem and academic achievement, overall life satisfaction, and happiness. However, the exact nature of this relationship is quite nuanced and often difficult to interpret. In particular, the relationship between self-esteem and academic performance is complex, and the direction of the relationship is unclear. For instance, does self-esteem lead to better grades, or does getting good grades lead to improved self-esteem? Most researchers agree today that the relationship is reciprocal (Baumeister et al., 2005). Furthermore, attempts to establish causality between self-esteem and various life outcomes via experimental or longitudinal studies have been largely unfruitful, and have suggested that self-esteem may be a byproduct of success rather than a cause (Baumeister et al., 2005; Forsyth & Kerr, 1999). One major study published at the end of the 1970s, when self-esteem-boosting programs were abundant in American schools (Scheirer & Kraut, 1979), found no causal link between popular self-esteem interventions and academic outcomes. Research has also produced conflicting, and sometimes surprising, results when examining the relationship between self-esteem and other outcomes. For instance, these studies have demonstrated that high self-esteem is positively correlated with various undesirable outcomes such as teen alcohol consumption, risky sexual behaviors, bullying, and delinquent behaviors (Baumeister et al., 2005). These studies found that teens with an inflated sense of self, or very high self-esteem, tend to engage in maladaptive behaviors just as frequently, and sometimes even more so, than their peers with lower self-esteem. Further complicating the research on the link between self-esteem and interpersonal variables is the fact that people with high self-esteem tend to inflate or exaggerate their abilities, skills, and popularity relative to people with lower self-esteem. As such, studies using self-report measures tend to yield strong positive correlations between self-esteem and interpersonal variables, but those results are often not replicated in studies that use direct observations, or parent, teacher, and peer ratings (Baumeister et al., 2003).

Many teachers and school children of the 1980s were inundated with various self-esteem activities designed to boost student's self-worth and teachers were frequently implored to lavish copious amounts of unconditional praise on their students to raise their self-esteem. However, subsequent research on praise and self-esteem has indicated this strategy of delivering effusive, inflated, and unconditional praise may backfire (Brummelman et al., 2014a, 2014b; Dweck, 2006). Two studies by Brummelman et al. (2013, 2014a, 2014b) found that providing inflated praise to children with low self-esteem (e.g., "that's the best drawing I've ever seen!") and praising personal qualities (e.g., intelligence), rather than praising process qualities (e.g., behavior or effort) may have deleterious effects on children with low self-esteem. Similarly, other researchers have cautioned that indiscriminate praise can have a detrimental effect on children (Dweck, 2006). For instance, praising fixed personal qualities, such as intelligence, seems to be a double-edged sword in that it gives children a short burst of pride in their intelligence, but then leads to a series of negative outcomes. For instance, students praised for their intelligence (in an effort to retain their status as "intelligent") tend to choose easy tasks to ensure success, are afraid of failure, afraid to ask for help, and strive to conceal their mistakes from others. They view effort as a sign of low intelligence and consequently, often pretend that tasks are easy and rush through them or are afraid to exert effort on tasks in front of other children. Furthermore, when they do fail it is a substantial blow to their self-esteem and their subsequent motivation to perform tasks suffers. In contrast, praising process (effort, persistence, engagement, etc.) rather than personal qualities improved motivation and enhanced subsequent performance.

By the 1990s, the self-esteem movement was already being widely mocked and parodied in popular culture, and it achieved the dreaded "eye-roll" status in society. Nothing epitomized this better than a popular skit created by Saturday Night Live involving a fictional self-help guru named Stuart Smalley. The sketch involved Stuart as the host of the talk show, "Daily Affirmations" where he would help boost the self-esteem of various celebrity guests with his self-affirming mantra: "I'm good enough, I'm smart enough, and doggone it, people like me!"

In the end, the failure of the self-esteem movement was not its proponent's belief in the importance of self-esteem. In fact, research has indicated that self-esteem is an important aspect of development and is correlated with several important outcomes such as happiness, and overall well-being. Instead, the failure of the self-esteem movement in schools can be attributed to the misinterpretation (and exploitation) of research and the exaggerated (and unequivocal) claims of zealots in the self-esteem movement who promoted the view that self-esteem was the cause of academic performance without considering that it might instead be the result of successful academic performance. Indeed, advocates employed a hallmark of "research based" pseudoscience practice advocacy, attributing causation to correlation. In the end, time was not on the side of the self-esteem movement, and it eventually withered under the spotlight proponents had created for it. Like most pseudoscience practices, the strategies and activities offered by proponents of the self-esteem movement were ultimately rejected by practitioners, and the general public at large, as the sheer ineffectiveness of the practices became readily apparent.

Open Classrooms

Open classrooms, also known as "schools without walls," were popular in America during the 1970s. The open classroom concept emerged from the open education reform movement of the 1960s (Barth & Rathbone, 1969; Barth, 1971) that was inspired by the "Informal Education" movement popular in England in the decades following World War II. At the time, the American public education system had been under serious attack by critics on both the left and right sides of the political spectrum. The prevailing sentiment in the country was that a major transformation of public education was crucial and long overdue. Critics on the political right blamed schools for several societal ills, including crime, urban decay, substance abuse, and even for America potentially losing the Cold War with the Soviet Union, whereas critics on the left attributed deteriorating student performance to schools' perpetuation of authoritarian and anti-quated educational practices (Cuban, 2004). The result was a perfect storm for change in a period of American history where the population was already inclined to challenge the status quo and question established societal norms. This provided a fertile environment for the open classroom movement to flourish.

The open classroom concept was based on the assumption that learners have the capacity to direct their own learning, and they should not be restricted by the barriers of traditional education (Barth & Rathbone, 1969; Barth, 1971; Cuban, 2004). Open classroom proponents emphasized that all students have the innate ability to learn on their own, that knowledge is constructed, that learning is a social process, and that students should be encouraged to learn and explore their environment independently. No detailed curriculum or whole class lessons were used, and standardized testing was rejected. The main goal of open classroom concept was to create an environment that was responsive to the needs of the students, allowing them to interact freely with their peers and work together to solve problems. The physical structure of the classroom was an integral component of learning in the open classroom concept. As such, classroom walls were physically removed from school buildings to create more flexible learning environments where students (and teachers) could work collaboratively on projects, in a multi-grade setting, and explore their interests at their own pace.

Without a shred of empirical evidence to support its effectiveness, the open classroom concept spread like a wildfire across the American educational landscape. By the middle of the 1970s, thousands of elementary school buildings across America were constructed or reno-vated (and countless millions of dollars were spent) to embody the "classrooms without walls" principle of the open classroom concept

(Cuban, 2004). Proponents believed that it was money well spent as they hypothesized that open classrooms would promote more effective student engagement, result in fewer behavioral issues, and substantially improve student achievement. Not surprisingly, these claims were not supported by subsequent research, and the once positive attitudes of administrators, teachers, students, and parents toward open classrooms shifted dramatically by the end of the decade.

In practice, the open classroom concept did not produce the promised results and problems emerged almost as quickly as the walls were being removed. Research studies failed to demonstrate that students in open classrooms performed better than traditional classrooms, and some studies indicated that it had a deleterious impact on performance (Henderson & Maddux, 1982; Horwitz, 1979). However, much of the research was wrought with methodological problems related to several issues. One major issue that researchers dealt with at the time was simply trying to determine and agree upon an operational definition of the term "open," or the degree to which a particular classroom was "open" and following the principles of open education (Rothenberg, 1989). In other words, schools across America were implementing their own interpretation of an "open classroom" and consequently, there was little consistency across districts or even within school districts. This inconsistency in implementation standards made it difficult for both researchers and teachers alike.

Collectively, much of the research conducted throughout the 1970s revealed no significant differences in academic achievement between students in open classrooms versus students in traditional classroom (Horwitz, 1979). However, the death knell for open classrooms was not just the research on poor academic outcomes, it was the views and attitudes of parents, teachers, and administrators, which had shifted dramatically against open classrooms by the end of the 1970s. Research on attitudes toward open classrooms revealed common complaints, such as increased student distraction, lack of student engagement, and an increasingly difficult and challenging teaching and learning environment (Henderson & Maddux, 1982; Rothenberg, 1989). Teachers and parents believed that the wide-open physical environment led to chaos and confusion for many students who struggled to focus and stay on task in the noisy environment of the open classroom. Not surprisingly, teachers in these studies frequently complained that they were not adequately trained or prepared to implement the open classroom concept and that the lack of a structured learning environment led to a substantial increase in behavior problems.

In response to criticism of the physical environment, many schools implemented design modifications in open classrooms that did appear to improve outcomes. One study (Evans & Lovell, 1979) investigated the effects of introducing acoustic and visual barriers (i.e., cleverly placed bookcases and sliding wall partitioners that could be opened and closed to separate groups) on the students' academic performance, behavior, and overall satisfaction. The results showed that the design modifications had a positive impact on the students, specifically enhancing their concentration and reducing distraction levels, leading to improved academic outcomes and higher satisfaction levels. These thin, accordion-style folding wall partitioners were a common feature in many classrooms throughout the 1980s and 1990s, though the walls themselves were rarely opened, resulting in a more traditional classroom experience for students and teachers.

Perhaps one lesson learned from the open classroom movement is the fact that an environment that is a fertile ground for change, is also fertile ground for pseudoscience practices. At the time the movement reached America, the public education system had been under intense public scrutiny and criticism. Waves of change are a common theme in educational history, but the wave of change that hit the American shoreline in the form of the open classroom movement was a veritable pseudoscience tsunami.

Summary and Conclusion

Historical pseudoscience practices in schools have had a significant impact on students. The pseudoscience practices reviewed in this chapter were often presented as reasonable, or even innovative, ideas that leveraged the zeitgeist of popular culture (e.g., open classrooms and the self-esteem movement) or simply served as the embodiment of misguided cultural beliefs (e.g., forced handedness and dunce caps). All were once widely accepted in schools, and by society at large. Most were replaced by more effective evidence-based practices, but in some cases, they were replaced by other pseudoscience practices. Some of these practices were presented as research based, but the research results were often misinterpreted or misrepresented by zealous proponents of the practice. All these practices lacked rigorous research support and empirical validation, but they often served to fill gaps in knowledge or to address a perceived need or weakness in education. Bias and poor clinical judgment often reside within these gaps in knowledge and thrive in ambiguity. The same is true for pseudoscience practices which often serve to fill these same knowledge gaps with practices that seem reasonable and well thought out. They often seem to scratch an itch in our change-centric field, but they lack solid empirical support and result in ineffectual services for the children in the greatest need. It is imperative that we blend innovation with critical analysis and continue to critically evaluate educational practices with research based on solid empirical evidence.

References

Alhassan, A. B. (2017). Left handedness, The Bible and The Quran: Implications for parents and teachers. *Research & Reviews: Journal of Educational Studies, 3*(1), 19–26.

Barth, R. S. (1971). So you want to change to an open classroom. *The Phi Delta Kappa, 53*(2), 97–99. Retrieved from http://www.jstor.org/stable/20373091

Barth, S., & Rathbone, C. H. (1969). *The open school: A way of thinking about children, learning, and knowledge.* Paper presented at the Center Forum.

Baumeister, R. F., Campbell, J. D., Krueger, J. I., & Vohs, K. D. (2003). Does High Self-Esteem Cause Better Performance, Interpersonal Success, Happiness, or Healthier Lifestyles? *Psychological Science in the Public Interest, 4*(1), 1–44.

Baumeister, R. F., Campbell, J. D., Krueger, J. I., & Vohs, K. D. (2005). Exploding the self-esteem myth. *Scientific American, 292*(1), 84–91. Retrieved from http://www.jstor.org/stable/26060842

Branden, N. (1984). In defense of self. *Association for Humanistic Psychology Newsletter,* 12–13.

Branden, N. (2001). *The psychology of self-esteem: A revolutionary approach to self-understanding that launched a new era in modern psychology: Thirty-second anniversary edition.* San Francisco: Jossey-Bass, 2001.

Brummelman, E., Thomaes, S., Orobio de Castro, B., Overbeek, G., & Bushman, B. J. (2014a). "That's Not Just Beautiful—That's Incredibly Beautiful!": The adverse impact of inflated praise on children with low self-esteem. *Psychological Science, 25*(3), 728–735. 10.1177/0956797613514251

Brummelman, E., Thomaes, S., Overbeek, G., Orobio de Castro, B., Van Den Hout, M. A., & Bushman, B. J. (2014b). On feeding those hungry for praise: Person praise backfires in children with low self-esteem. *Journal of Experimental Psychology: General, 143*(1), 9.

Cuban, L. (2004). The open classroom: Were schools without walls just another fad? *Education Next, 4*(2), 68–72.

Diener, E., & Diener, M. (1995). Cross-cultural correlates of life satisfaction and self-esteem. *Journal of Personality and Social Psychology, 68*(4), 653–663.

Dweck, C. S. (2006). *Mindset: The new psychology of success.* New York: Random House

Evans, G. W., & Lovell, B. (1979). Design modification in an open-plan school. *Journal of Educational Psychology, 71*(1), 41.

Forsyth, D., & Kerr, N. (1999). *Are adaptive illusions adaptive.* Paper presented at the Poster presented at the annual meeting of the American Psychological Association, Boston, MA.

Hansford, B. C., & Hattie, J. A. (1982). The relationship between self and achievement/performance measures. *Review of Educational Research, 52*(1), 123–142. doi:10.3102/00346543052001123

Henderson, D. L., & Maddux, C. D. (1982). Open-concept schools: Popularity, disillusionment, and attitudes. *Education, 103*(2), 183–185.

Horwitz, R. A. (1979). Psychological effects of the "Open Classroom". *Review of Educational Research, 49*(1), 71–85. doi:10.3102/00346543049001071

Klein, D. C. (1991). The humiliation dynamic: An overview. *Journal of Primary Prevention*, *12*(2), 93–121. doi:10.1007/BF02015214

Klöppel, S., Mangin, J. F., Vongerichten, A., Frackowiak, R. S., & Siebner, H. R. (2010). Nurture versus nature: Long-term impact of forced right-handedness on structure of pericentral cortex and basal ganglia. *Journal of Neuroscience*, *30*(9), 3271–3275. doi:10.1523/jneurosci.4394-09.2010

McManus, C. (2019). Half a century of handedness research: Myths, truths; fictions, facts; backwards, but mostly forwards. *Brain and Neuroscience Advances*, *3*, 2398212818820513. doi:10.1177/2398212818820513

Mecca, A., Smelser, N. J., & Vasconcellos, J. (1989). *The social importance of self-esteem*. Univ of California Press.

Porac, C. (2016). *Laterality: Exploring the enigma of left-handedness*. New York: Academic Press.

Pottebaum, S. M., Keith, T. Z., & Ehly, S. W. (1986). Is there a causal relation between self-concept and academic achievement? *The Journal of Educational Research*, *79*(3), 140–144. doi:10.1080/00220671.1986.10885665

Rothenberg, J. (1989). The open classroom reconsidered. *The Elementary School Journal*, *90*(1), 69–86. doi:10.1086/461603

Scheirer, M. A., & Kraut, R. E. (1979). Increasing educational achievement via self-concept change. *Review of Educational Research*, *49*(1), 131–149.

Sha, Z., Pepe, A., Schijven, D., Carrión-Castillo, A., Roe, J. M., Westerhausen, R., … Francks, C. (2021). Handedness and its genetic influences are associated with structural asymmetries of the cerebral cortex in 31,864 individuals. *Proceedings of the National Academy of Sciences of United States of America*, *118*(47), e2113095118. doi:10.1073/pnas.2113095118

Singal, J. (2017). How the self-esteem craze took over America and why the hype was irresistible. Retrieved from https://www.thecut.com/2017/05/self-esteem-grit-do-they-really-help.html Stephen Hupp 11-Jan-2024 20:26 Retrieved from https://www.thecut.com/2017/05/self-esteem-grit-do-they-really-help.html

Stearns, P. N., & Stearns, C. (2017). American schools and the uses of shame: An ambiguous history. *History of Education*, *46*(1), 58–75. doi:10.1080/0046760X.2016.1185671

Terman. (1914). *The hygiene of the school child*. Boston: Houghton Mifflin.

Weaver, H. A. (2012). Object lessons: A cultural genealogy of the dunce cap and the apple as visual tropes of American education. *Paedagogica Historica*, *48*(2), 215–241. doi:10.1080/00309230.2011.560856

Part II
Systems-level Practices

3 Zero-Tolerance Policies

Angela Fontanini-Axelrod

School safety has become a serious concern for parents, educators, and students in the United States. For example, a 2022 Gallup poll reported that 44% of parents expressed fear for their oldest child's physical safety at school, representing a 10% increase from 2019 (Brenan, 2022). That same poll found students' fear about school safety is the highest they have been in over 20 years. Increased threats to school safety have led to increased focus on school security and disciplinary practices (see Mowen & Freng, 2019). For the last 30 years, school security and discipline have been dominated by the philosophy of zero tolerance. The term "zero tolerance" dates to the 1980s with the federal government's "war on drugs"; in 1994, the Gun-Free Schools Act was passed, mandating out-of-school suspension for one year for any student with a weapon to school. It did not take long for the zero- tolerance philosophy and corresponding measures to be applied across a variety of other issues (e.g., environmental pollution, sexual harassment) including school discipline. While there is no singular definition of "zero-tolerance," these policies generally "mandate the application of predetermined consequences, most often severe and punitive in nature, that are intended to be applied regardless of the gravity of behavior, mitigating circumstances, or situational context" (APA Zero Tolerance Task Force, 2008, p. 852). Under zero-tolerance policies, school administrators employ consequences (e.g., suspension, expulsion) to punish rule violations (Welsh & Little, 2018).

This chapter focuses on three primary claims: 1) zero-tolerance policies can help make discipline decisions consistent across all students and have a deterrent effect, 2) zero-tolerance policies provide a positive school climate and supportive learning environment, and 3) parents and teachers consistently endorse zero-tolerance policies.

Examining the Claims

To fully examine zero-tolerance policies, it will be helpful to consider reasons why school personnel claim there is a need for these policies. School

DOI: 10.4324/9781003266181-5

shootings have occurred for decades; however, they increased notably in the 1990s (Carlton, 2017; Katsiyannis et al., 2018). Following the Columbine (Colorado) High School tragedy in 1999, the yearly occurrence of school shootings remained relatively stable until an increase in school shootings was observed again in 2015 (Cox et al., 2021; Gunfire on School Grounds in the United States, 2019; Parks et al., 2019). These events are undeniably tragic, and prevention of all school violence has understandably emerged as a top priority for all stakeholders. To combat school violence and ensure student safety, schools must have smart and effective discipline policies that are implemented fairly across students and infractions.

While school shootings are indeed a national tragedy and should receive media coverage, media attention given to shootings has the potential to bias our understanding of how common shootings happen at individual schools. Conventional wisdom and pop culture also tend to elevate fears. Television shows, for example, often sensationalize school violence – the HBO show "Euphoria" depicts a group of high school students who engage in heavy drug use and physical violence, and the popular Netflix series "13 Reasons Why" contains storylines involving regular instances of school violence, including a school shooting.

The Analysis of the School-Associated Violent Death Study reported that approximately two dozen school-age children in the United States are murdered every week, but only about 1% of those murders occur at school. Although any level of violence is unacceptable, evidence fails to support the claim that extreme violence is a high risk for any given school. Although there has been an increase in school shootings in the last decade, incidents of deadly violence remain a relatively small proportion of reported school violence, and data have consistently demonstrated that overall school violence has remained stable, or even decreased slightly, since approximately 1985.

As a response to these concerns, K-12 schools across the country have understandably engaged in efforts to prevent school violence. The results have been mixed. Approximately 67% of school districts employ mandatory expulsion policies for certain offenses (e.g., bringing a weapon to school); however, these expulsion policies have also been applied to an expanding definition of what constitutes a "weapon" and a range of student behaviors that do not involve a weapon such as classroom disruption or verbal aggression (Curran, 2019). Given these issues, claims related to school violence deserve a closer examination.

Claim 1: Zero-Tolerance Policies Make Discipline Decisions Consistent across All Students and Have a Deterrent Effect

Proponents of zero-tolerance policies often claim that utilizing a "one size fits all" approach brings fairness to disciplinary decisions, eliminating bias, and establishing clear consequences for student misbehavior. Initially, zero-tolerance policies were those that involved predetermined punishments for specific categories of serious misbehavior (for example, bringing a weapon to school or distributing illegal drugs at school). However, zero tolerance has transformed into a broad set of punitive disciplinary practices that exclude children from learning for a range of misbehaviors including those considered somewhat minor or trivial (for example, being disrespectful to a teacher). Zero tolerance for firearms expanded to the general approach of automatically expelling or suspending students for an increasingly wide range of rule violations and circumstances, even if the behavior was unintentional or posed no serious threat to others such as a student who forgot to take his Boy Scout knife out of his backpack after a camping trip. This "consistency" has resulted in school administrators viewing all violations, from simple misunderstandings and social gaffes to willful wrongdoing, as equally serious when judged according to zero-tolerance philosophy.

Consistency is an important criterion in the implementation of any school discipline policy. Yet, there is no evidence that zero-tolerance policies improve the consistency of how discipline is implemented (APA Zero Tolerance Task Force, 2008). Discipline practices can differ greatly across schools and districts, and differences appear to be as much a characteristic of schools and personnel (e.g., disciplinary philosophy, effective school leaders) as the behavior of students. Punitive disciplinary practices, including and especially zero-tolerance policies, have led to systemic racism in schools. Biases and prejudice influence subjective interpretations of behavior as well as the selection and implementation of disciplinary practices (Henry et al., 2022).

Unfortunately, schools have also implemented zero-tolerance policies that punish students for minor infractions, hoping this will deter other students from engaging in more serious misbehavior (Borum et al., 2010). Most often these expulsions and suspensions for minor infractions involve overreactions by school staff or misunderstandings. For example, a high school student brought apples to school for a "healthy eating" presentation and cut them with a knife, only to learn later he was suspended for bringing a weapon to school. Also, an eight-year-old student bit his pastry into the shape of a gun and was suspended. Similarly, a second-grader was suspended for pointing a pencil playfully at a friend and adding gun noises (McNamara, 2013). Again, zero-tolerance policies have expanded the view of what constitutes a weapon and, in an effort to create more consistent disciplinary responses to rule infractions, have lead school administrators to overreact in the name of zero tolerance.

Proponents argue that these policies are part of the solution to dealing with safety issues because they serve to deter future misbehavior (see Bishop & Feld, 2012; Gottfredson, 2017). School administrators claim that cracking down on small offenses makes students feel safer and discourages more serious rule violations, and this results in suspensions for offenses that were previously met with disciplinary reactions like detentions. However, the effectiveness of these policies in preventing such problems has not been established (Reeping et al., 2021). For example, research by the American Psychological Association has suggested that such policies and practices likely negatively impact students' educational experience without any noteworthy improvement in the safety of the school environment (Skiba & Sprague, 2008). Moreover, zero-tolerance policies and practices fail to effectively attend to systemic causes of students' problems and likely lead to more disruption than benefit (Teske, 2011). Expulsion is associated with higher dropout rates and delayed graduation, and the ACLU (2008) reports that zero-tolerance policies result in significant increases in expulsions and suspensions. Furthermore, researchers have concluded that suspension does not effectively improve student behavior, as students often return to school exhibiting the same or even more severe behavior (Skiba, 2000), and psychologists have regularly stated concerns that zero-tolerance policies have the potential to criminalize students (Borum et al., 2010).

School professionals themselves often do not see the efficacy of these policies in deterring violence and misbehavior. In a study examining school professionals' experience with zero-tolerance policies in their schools, more than half indicated that zero-tolerance policies did not work well in schools (Henry et al., 2022). Most teachers either disagreed or strongly disagreed with the idea that zero-tolerance policies make schools safer or more effective in handling disciplinary issues. Taken together, this evidence refutes the claim that zero-tolerance policies maintain consistency in discipline and have a deterrent effect.

Claim 2: Zero-Tolerance Policies Provide a Positive School Climate and Supportive Learning Environment

Proponents of zero-tolerance policies claim that tough responses to student misbehavior assist in providing a positive and supportive school environment. Although the assumption might make sense intuitively, data from several indicators have shown the opposite effect. Specifically, research suggests that higher rates of school suspension and expulsion are associated with low ratings of school climate. Over a decade ago, the APA Zero Tolerance Task Force (2008) could find no scientific support for the claim that zero-tolerance policies improved school climate or school safety. If zero-tolerance policies are effective, schools that approach discipline from a zero-tolerance perspective would presumably have fewer students engaging in disruptive behaviors and both students and staff should report feeling safe. However, zero-tolerance policies predict negative outcomes including school disengagement, dropout, repeating a grade, criminal justice involvement, problems with substance use, and student trauma (Skiba & Noam, 2001; Teasley & Miller, 2011).

Research shows a negative relationship between suspensions/expulsions and schoolwide academic achievement, even when controlling for demographic variables. For example, Lee et al. (2011) found that dropout rates are significantly more common for schools that suspended over one-fifth of their students compared to schools that suspended less than 10%. Furthermore, high school students given out-of-school suspensions or expulsions are considerably more likely to eventually drop out of school (Lamont et al., 2013). The ACLU report also noted a recognized trend indicating a relationship between high rates of school suspension and high school dropout numbers. The ACLU reported nearly 50% of students starting high school with three or more suspensions eventually drop out of school (Balfanz et al., 2014). Although such correlational findings do not demonstrate causality, there is no evidence that zero-tolerance policies create more positive school environments when their use is associated with more negative educational outcomes.

In addition, research suggests that zero-tolerance policies and procedures are fundamentally biased toward underrepresented populations (Allen et al., 2013; Curran, 2016; Logan & Burdick-Will, 2017; Welsh & Little, 2018). Black students are more likely to receive exclusionary discipline at a disproportionately high rate. This pattern begins early; 48% of preschool children suspended more than once are Black (CRDC, 2014). The behaviors of Black students are often punished more severely and often lead to criminal justice system referrals (National Association of Education, 2020) and increased incarceration (Cruz & Rodl, 2018). Although Black students only make up 15% of the student population, they received about 39% of out-of-school suspensions (US Department of Education, 2019). The Civil Rights Data Collection (OCR, 2018) report that Black male students represent 8% of enrolled students yet account for 25% of students who receive at least one suspension. Research suggests exclusionary practices are not only disproportionately used in cases involving underrepresented students (e.g., students of color, students with disabilities) and male students (Riddle & Sinclair, 2019; Shabazian, 2015), but studies also indicate that these practices promote negative and potentially long-lasting consequences for students' educational, psychological, and social development (Adams et al., 2012; Crosby et al., 2018).

Zero-tolerance policies have also been shown to specifically impact Black females and Black children with disabilities. Research from the U.S.

Department of Education Office for Civil Rights reports that 12% of Black girls were suspended in the 2011–2012 school year compared to 2% for White girls (Civil Rights Snapshot, 2014). Moreover, almost 25% of Black boys with disabilities and 20% of Black girls with disabilities were suspended during the 2011–2012 school year. Advocacy groups, like the Center for Civil Rights Remedies, view these results as problematic because research has not found higher rates of weapon use in Black female or disabled populations.

A positive school climate is characterized by people feeling supported socially, emotionally, and physically. For school climate to truly be positive, all students must feel safe and supported. However, the evidence suggests zero-tolerance policies might create the opposite effect resulting in negative learning environments and poor outcomes for specific student populations, including students of color and students with disabilities.

Claim 3: Stakeholders Consistently Endorse Zero-Tolerance Policies

Proponents of zero-tolerance policies claim that parents, teachers, and other stakeholders support these types of disciplinary approaches. However, data indicating support for these policies among parents and teachers are mixed and inconclusive. Some research suggests that parents and community members support punitive disciplinary actions (e.g., expulsion, suspension) if student safety is threatened. The American Psychological Association Zero Tolerance Task Force (2008) reported that parents overwhelmingly support the implementation of zero-tolerance policies when their children's safety is at stake. Even beyond serious threats to student safety, zero-tolerance policies decrease parental concerns that less significant problem behavior (e.g., bullying, defiance) is dealt with swiftly and in no uncertain terms. Parents who support zero-tolerance policies erroneously believe that such disciplinary practices keep schools safe because these practices limit opportunities and encourage students to report problems (e.g., bullying behavior, presence of guns, weapons, and drugs) to school administrators. In addition, conventional wisdom suggests that some students may change their behaviors as a result of disciplinary actions brought on by zero-tolerance policies.

However, zero-tolerance policies are not always favored by stakeholder groups. For example, Henry et al. (2022) found that only 25% of parents surveyed believed that zero-tolerance policies had a positive effect on their children's school, whereas an equal number had indicated that zero-tolerance was a failed policy and, perhaps more importantly, had a negative effect. The authors noted that all participants indicating zero-tolerance policies were positive or very positive identified as White. Huang and Cornell (2021) reported that both students and teachers in schools that had greater support for zero-tolerance policies indicated feeling less safe at school, even after controlling for school and student characteristics associated with safety. The authors also noted finding no empirical studies showing an association between zero-tolerance policies in school and parent and student perceptions of safety. Students themselves regard school suspension as ineffective and unfair. McNeal and Dunbar (2010) found that students continued to feel unsafe in schools more than a decade after the policy's initiation.

Summary and Conclusions

The APA Zero Tolerance Task Force (2008), following an exhaustive review of the literature, concluded that stricter and overly punitive disciplinary policies do not make schools safer. Since the Task Force's report, research has found that zero-tolerance practices do not improve school safety but, in fact, promote further misbehavior and do nothing to increase academic achievement (Cornell et al., 2021). However, schools continue to adopt school safety procedures involving zero-tolerance policies for weapons, drugs, and other disciplinary infractions with the belief that these policies work to deter future offenders (see Teske, 2011). Furthermore, zero tolerance has been extended to address minor misbehavior including defiance (Skiba & Losen, 2015/2016). Zero-tolerance policies assume that disciplining students who engage in any type of problem behavior will discourage others and create improved learning environments (Ewing, 2000).

School violence and student safety should be top priorities and taken seriously. Furthermore, schools must have effective discipline policies that are implemented consistently across students and infractions. Given zero-tolerance policies have little to no empirical support and there are clearly many negative outcomes associated with punitive disciplinary policies and practices, numerous researchers and professional organizations have argued for policy changes with respect to school disciplinary practices and more thoughtful implementation of alternative discipline approaches in schools (Welsh & Little, 2018). Restorative justice and Positive Behavioral Interventions and Supports (PBIS) are two commonly employed school practices that take advantage of principles with strong empirical evidence. Restorative justice practices aim to facilitate positive interactions between the victim and the offender as a mechanism to address previous wrongdoing. The practice takes a proactive approach by facilitating the development of communication and relationship skills to reduce the prospect of future problems, which contrasts with a more reactive approach inherent to many exclusionary discipline practices (Dorado et al., 2016; Mansfield et al., 2018).

PBIS involves supporting students using behavioral approaches that both encourage and reinforce positive behavior (Swain-Bradway et al., 2015). Restorative justice and PBIS take situational circumstances and individual characteristics into account and emphasize fostering the development of alternative (prosocial and adaptive) behaviors. Furthermore, interventions emphasizing culturally sensitive learning, social-emotional learning, and teacher-student relationships have been more effective at reducing the prevalence of school-based violations when compared to punishment-focused policies (Welsh & Little, 2018).

Zero-tolerance policies have failed to realize the goals of an effective school discipline model. Zero tolerance has failed to demonstrate improved school climate or school safety and its application has not worked to improve student behavior. Furthermore, zero-tolerance policies have not resolved, and indeed may have exacerbated, the over-representation of students of color and students with disabilities in school discipline.

References

Adams, G. S., Mullen, E., & Guala, F. (2012). The social and psychological costs of punishing. *Behavioral and Brain Sciences*, 35(1), 15–16.

American Psychological Association Zero Tolerance Task Force (2008). Are zero-tolerance policies effective in the schools? An evidentiary review of recommendations. *The American Psychologist*, 63(9), 852–862.

Allen, A., Scott, L. M., & Lewis, C. W. (2013). Racial microaggressions and African American and Hispanic students in urban schools: A call for culturally affirming education. *Interdisciplinary Journal of Teaching and Learning*, 3(2), 117–129.

American Civil Liberties Union (ACLU) (2008). *Dignity denied: The effects of "zero tolerance" policies on students' human rights.* https://www.aclu.org/sites/default/files/pdfs/humanrights/dignitydenied_november2008.pdf

Balfanz, R., Byrnes, V., & Fox, J. (2014). Sent home and put off-track: The antecedents, disproportionalities, and consequences of being suspended in the ninth grade. *Journal of Applied Research on Children: Informing Policy for Children at Risk*, 5(2), Article 13.

Bishop, D. M., & Feld, B. C. (2012). Trends in juvenile justice policy and practice. In B. C. Feld & D. M. Bishop (Eds.), *The Oxford handbook of juvenile crime and juvenile justice* (pp. 898–926). Oxford University Press.

Borum, R., Cornell, D. G., Modzeleski, W., & Jimerson, S. R. (2010). What can be done about school shootings? *Educational Researcher*, 39(1), 27–37.

Brenan, M. (2022). Parent, student safety concerns elevated. Retrieved from https://news.gallup.com/poll/399680/parent-student-school-safety-concerns-elevated.aspx

Carlton, M. P. (2017). Summary of school safety statistics. National Institute of Justice Report, US Department of Justice.

Civil Rights Data Collection (2014). Data snapshot: School discipline. US Department of Education Office for Civil Rights Issue Brief No. 1.

Cornell, D., Mayer, M., & Sulkowski, M. (2021). History and future of school safety research. *School Psychology Review, 50*(2/3), 143–157.

Cox, J., Rich, S., Chiu, A., Muyskens, J., & Ulmanu, M. (2021). *More than 278,000 students have experienced gun violence at school since Columbine.* Washington Post. https://www.washingtonpost.com/graphics/2018/local/school-shootings-database/?utm_term=.c7bd3effe7e1.

Crosby, S., Howell, P., & Thomas, M. (2018). Social justice education through trauma-informed teaching. *Middle School Journal, 49,* 15–23.

Cruz, R. A., & Rodl, J. E. (2018). Crime and punishment: An examination of school context and student characteristics that predict out-of-school suspension. *Children & Youth Services Review, 95,* 226–234.

Curran, F. C. (2019). The Law, Policy, and Portrayal of Zero Tolerance School Discipline: Examining Prevalence and Characteristics Across Levels of Governance and School Districts. *Educational Policy, 33*(2), 319–349.

Curran, F. C. (2016). Estimating the effect of state zero tolerance laws on exclusionary discipline, racial discipline gaps, and student behavior. *Educational Evaluation and Policy Analysis, 38,* 647–668.

Dorado, J., Martinez, M., McArthur, L., & Leibovitz, T. (2016). Healthy Environments and Response to Trauma in Schools (HEARTS): A whole-school, multi-level, prevention and intervention program for creating trauma-informed, safe and supportive schools. *School Mental Health, 8,* 163–176. Available at: 10.1007/s12310-016-9177-0

Ewing, C. P. (2000, January/February). *Sensible zero tolerance protects students.* Harvard Education Letter. https://digitalcommons.law.buffalo.edu/journal_articles/504

Gottfredson, D. C. (2017). Prevention research in schools: Past, present, and future. *American Society of Criminology, 16,* 1–21.

Gunfire on School Grounds in the United States (2019). *Everytown for gun safety.* https://everytownresearch.org/gunfire-in-school/#16181

Henry, K. K., Catagnus, R. M., Griffith, A. K., & Garcia, Y. A. (2022). Ending the school-to-prison pipeline: Perception and experience with zero-tolerance policies and interventions to address racial inequality. *Behavior Analysis in Practice, 15,* 1254–1263.

Huang, F. & Cornell, D. (2021). Teacher support for zero tolerance is associated with higher suspension rates and lower feelings of safety. *School Psychology Review, 50*(2–3), 388–405.

Katsiyannis, A., Whitford, D., Ennis, R. (2018). Historical examination of United States intentional mass school shootings in the 20th and 21st centuries: Implications for students, schools, and society. *Journal of Child and Family Studies, 27,* 2562–2573.

Lamont, J. H., Devore, C. D., Allison, M., Ancona, R., Barnett, S. E., Gunther, R., Holmes, B., Minier, M., Okamoto, J. K., Wheller, L. S. M., & Young, T. (2013). Out-of-school suspension and expulsion. *Pediatrics, 131* (3), 1000–1007.

Lee, T., Cornell, D., Gregory, A., & Fan, X. (2011). High suspension schools and dropout rates for black and white students. *Education and Treatment of Children, 34*(2), 167–192.

Logan, J. R., & Burdick-Will, J. (2017). School segregation and disparities in urban, suburban, and rural areas. *The Annals of the American Academy of Political and Social Science, 674*, 199–216.

Mansfield, K. C., Fowler, B., & Rainbolt, S. (2018). The potential of restorative practices to ameliorate discipline gaps: The story of one high school's leadership team. *Educational Administration Quarterly., 54*(2), 303–323.

McNamara, A. (2013, May 9). *Boy suspended after pretending pencil is a gun.* NBC News. Retrieved from https://www.nbcnews.com/ watch/nbc-news-channel/boy-suspended-after-pretendingpencil-is-a-gun-44443203985

McNeal, L., & Dunbar, C. J. (2010) In the eyes of the beholder: Urban students' perception of zero tolerance policy. *Urban Education, 45*(3), 293–311.

Mowen, T. J., & Freng, A. (2019). Is more necessarily better? School security and perceptions of safety among students and parents in the United States. *American Journal of Criminal Justice, 44*(3), 376–394.

National Association of Education (2020). Building relationship and community to prevent and address conflict: Ending the school to prison pipeline. https://neaedjustice.org/ending-the-school-to-prison-pipeline/

Office of Civil Rights (2018). Data on equal access to education. Civil Rights Data Collection.

Parks, J., Bechtold, D., Shelp, F., Lieberman, J., & Coffey, S. (2019). *Mass violence in America: Causes, impacts and solutions.* https://www.thenationalcouncil.org/wp-content/uploads/2019/08/Mass-Violence-in-America_8-6-19.pdf?daf=375ateTbd56

Reeping, P. M., Gobaud, A., Branas, C. C., & Rajan, S. (2021). K–12 school shootings: Implications for policy, prevention, and child well-being. *Pediatric Clinics of North America, 68*(2), 413–426.

Riddle, T., & Sinclair, S. (2019). Racial disparities in school-based disciplinary actions are associated with county-level rates of racial bias. *Proceedings of the National Academy of Sciences of the United States of America, 116*(17), 8255–8260.

School-Associated Violent Death Study. (2019). *Centers for disease control and prevention.* https://www.cdc.gov/violenceprevention/youthviolence/schoolviolence/SAVD.html

Shabazian A. N. (2015). The significance of location: Patterns of school exclusionary disciplinary practices in public schools. *Journal of School Violence, 14*(3), 273–298.

Skiba, R. (2000). *Zero tolerance, zero evidence: An analysis of school discipline practice.* Bloomington: Indiana University Education Policy Center.

Skiba, R. J., & Losen, D. (2015/2016). From reaction to prevention: Turning the page on school discipline. *American Educator, 39*, 4–11.

Skiba, R. J., & Noam, G. G. (2001). *Zero tolerance: Can suspension and expulsion keep schools safe?* Jossey-Bass.

Skiba, R., & Sprague, J. (2008). Safety without suspensions. *Educational Leadership, 66*(1), 38–43.

Swain-Bradway, J., Pinkney, C., & Flannery, K. B. (2015). Implementing schoolwide positive behavior interventions and supports in high schools: Contextual factors and stages of implementation. *Teaching Exceptional Children, 47*(5), 245–255.

Teasley, M. I., & Miller, C. (2011). School social workers' perceived efficiency at tasks related to curbing suspensions and undesirable behaviors. *Children & Schools, 33*, 136–145.

Teske, S. C. (2011). A study of zero tolerance policies in schools: A multi-integrated systems approach to improve outcomes for adolescents. *Journal of Child and Adolescent Psychiatric Nursing, 24*, 88–97.

U.S. Department of Education (2019). The Condition of Education. National Center for Educational Statistics.

Welsh, R. O., & Little, S. (2018). Caste and control in schools: A systematic review of the pathways, rates, and correlates of exclusion due to school discipline. *Children and Youth Services Review, 94*, 315–339.

4 Suicide Prevention and Intervention Practices

Susan M. Swearer, Samantha Kesselring, and Emilea Rejman

Youth suicide is a public health crisis that plagues the United States. According to the Centers for Disease Control (CDC, 2019), suicide ranks as one of the leading causes of death among teens. Compounding this situation, in the United States alone, suicide rates have dramatically increased over the past several decades (Curtin, 2020; McKeown et al., 2006), with a significant increase in youth suicide during the COVID-19 pandemic (Bridge et al., 2023). Youth spend most of their days in schools; therefore, school-based prevention and intervention programs are vital for reducing youth suicide rates. It is critical that prevention and intervention efforts are evaluated to understand the benefits and limitations of current programming and to promote evidence-based suicide prevention and intervention. This chapter will introduce eight misconceptions about youth suicide and will examine each from an empirical perspective. Finally, we offer some guidance on what school personnel can do to address suicide from both prevention and intervention perspectives.

Examining the Claims

Claim #1: Suicide Attempters and Completers Are Similar

There are many common misconceptions about youth suicide that arise from a lack of understanding about depression and suicide. The first misconception is that suicide attempters and completers are similar (Moskos et al., 2004). Research has found that there are differences across gender identity, race, and age between suicide completers and attempters (e.g., Cai et al., 2021; Kreski et al., 2022; Schmutte & Wilkinson, 2020). Globally, the gender difference in suicide completion tends to be 1.8 times higher for males than females (World Health Organization, 2019). Suicide completers tend to be more likely male than female (Cibis et al., 2012); however, females have higher rates of suicide attempts (Cai et al., 2021; Kaess et al., 2011; Weissman et al., 1999). Differences in method have also been explored (Callanan & Davis, 2012;

DOI: 10.4324/9781003266181-6

Denning et al., 2000; Värnik et al., 2008). Cai et al. (2021) examined whether choice of method differed across genders. Roughly 62.4% of the greater number of male suicides were explained by access to firearms (Cai et al., 2021). Importantly, suicide *attempts* tend to be highest among adolescents (Schmutte & Wilkinson, 2020).

Claim #2: Teens Have the Highest Suicide Rate

Teens having the highest *completed* suicides is another common misconception (Moskos et al., 2004). According to the CDC (2019), the highest suicide rate is among adults between the ages of 55 and 64. While suicide is a leading cause of death among teens (CDC, 2019), compared to other age groups, teens do not rank highest in number of suicides. Suicide has been linked to family and social stress (Moskos et al, 2004). Conflict within the family structure has also been linked to suicide among teens (Daniel & Goldston, 2009). While teen suicide is not directly caused by familial stress, a range of multiple factors contribute to teen suicide including biological, environmental, psychological, and social factors (Moskos et al., 2004). Thus, it is of the utmost importance to use comprehensive screening procedures that include questions about family history and environmental stressors and refer them to appropriate mental health resources (Moskos et al., 2004).

Claim #3: Talking about Suicide Will Promote Suicidal Behavior

Another misconception is that talking about suicide will promote suicidal behavior (Mazza, 1997). This simply is not the case, and talking about depression and suicidal ideation has been shown to help individuals who are thinking about self-harm and suicide. Research has shown that discussing suicide for a person at-risk of attempting suicide aids in decreasing the likelihood of a suicide attempt and allows for discussion regarding why the individual may be feeling this way (Pérez Barrero & Sereno Batista, 2001; Pérez Barrero, 2003; Reynolds, 1988; Reynolds & Mazza, 1994). Despite this research finding, it is important to consider suicide contagion effects when discussing suicide (Berman et al., 2006; Gould & Davidson, 1988). A suicide cluster is identified when suicides occur in short periods of time and in close geographical proximity than is typically expected for a specific area (CDC, 1988). Gould and Lake (2013) state that up to 5% of adolescent suicides occur in a cluster following another youth dying by suicide. Guidelines have been released as a preventative strategy to reduce the likelihood of suicide clusters. The World Health Organization recommends that media outlets not share nor repeat the story; graphic depictions should not be shared; and specific details about the lethal method used should not be reported. The National Association for School Psychologists (NASP) has also issued guidelines to help avoid contagion including confirming the facts, calling in a crisis response team, monitoring at-risk students, informing the students personally, giving opportunity for proper mental health support, and community engagement and involvement (Zenere, 2009).

Claim #4: Teen Suicide Is Primarily a Result of Treatment Failure

Teen suicide is a result of treatment failure is another common misconception (Moskos et al., 2004). Rowe et al. (2014) found that most individuals exhibiting suicide-related behaviors do not seek treatment. Between 30% and 45% seek help from professionals following an attempted suicide (Slovak & Singer, 2012; Wu et al., 2010). Among those who seek help, nearly half drop out of treatment (Brent et al., 2013; Glenn et al., 2015; Simes et al., 2022). Since previous suicide attempts are the leading risk factor for completed suicides (Franklin et al., 2017), treatment for suicide attempters is critical.

Claim #5: Prevention Programs Are Sufficient in Preventing Youth Suicide

There is a misconception that prevention programs are sufficient in preventing youth suicide (Moskos et al., 2004). While current prevention programs are better than no programming, many prevention programs do not have a sufficient evidence base. The literature regarding suicide prevention and intervention reviews several programs including, but not limited to (1) gatekeeper training (e.g., Question, Persuade and Refer [QPR]) and (2) psychoeducational and peer leadership training (e.g., Sources of Strength; Care, Assess, Respond, Empower [CARE]), Coping and Support Training [CAST], Reconnecting Youth [RY], and the Good Behavior Game [GBG]; Katz et al., 2013). These programs are promising; however, no singular intervention is considered the "gold standard" (Katz et al., 2013; Kong et al., 2016). There is an urgent need for more randomized controlled trials evaluating the efficacy of these programs (Bennett et al., 2015; Brann et al., 2021; Breet et al., 2021; Brown et al., 2007; Katz et al., 2013; Miller & Emanuele, 2009; Robinson et al., 2013). Research in suicide prevention and intervention is at a critical turning point. While evaluating what works, what doesn't work, and what can work better, it is critical to address the deficiencies in suicide prevention programming. Several empirical reviews confirm that current programs are simply not enough (Bennett et al., 2015; Cusimano & Sameem, 2011; Katz et al., 2013; Kong et al., 2016).

Claim #6: Intervention Programs Are Universally Effective

Suicide prevention strategies can be categorized by their outreach. There are three different levels of outreach discussed in the literature; universal, selected, and indicated. Universal prevention strategies are designed to reach all students. These programs enhance awareness, provide resources on where to seek help, teach helping and coping skills and ways for individuals to provide support to one another, reduce stigma, and empower students to seek help (Bailey et al., 2017; Breet et al., 2021). Comprehensive universal suicide prevention and intervention programs have been used to educate individuals on the risk factors and warning signs, expand knowledge about intervention and prevention practices, discuss misperceptions about suicide, respond appropriately to those indicating suicidal ideation, and recognize students who may be at-risk for suicidal ideation or may currently be suicidal (Mazza & Reynolds, 2008; Miller & Emanuele 2009). Criticisms of universal prevention programs include the brevity of programs and the lack of focus on psychoeducation (Berman et al., 2006; Kalafat, 2003; Mazza, 1997; Miller & Emanuele, 2009; Miller & DuPaul, 1996). According to Miller & Emanuele (2009), a large portion of universal prevention programs are directed at teaching curriculum to students. Although Zenere and Lazarus (1997) demonstrated longevity of a 5-year plan to educate students, Miller and Emanuele (2009) found that most universal programs are yielding weak evidence.

Selective prevention strategies are aimed at students at higher risk of suicide (Hill & Pettit, 2019). One prevention strategy that is commonly implemented is gatekeeper training. Gatekeepers refer to individuals (i.e., administrators, staff, and peers) who can aid in helping youth who are at-risk. Gatekeeper training involves educating these individuals to recognize the warning signs, provide support to at-risk students, know how and where to access help, and feel empowered to act (Breet et al., 2021). QPR is a gatekeeper training that focuses on four important steps: (1) identifying warning signs, (2) training staff, (3) training counselors to assess students at-risk, and (4) providing treatment (QPR Institute, 2011). Yet, some flaws have been found with only using gatekeeper training. Specifically, QPR Institute (2011) found that only gatekeepers who felt comfortable and confident in their abilities approached students to get them the help they needed.

Claim #7: There Is a "Gold Standard" in Suicide Prevention and Intervention

Katz et al. (2013) conducted an extensive systematic review of 16 school-based suicide prevention programs. Importantly, many programs were aimed at improving knowledge and attitudes surrounding suicide, not reducing suicide attempts (Cusimano & Sameem, 2011; Katz et al., 2013).

Only two programs, Signs of Suicide (SOS) and the Good Behavior Game (GBG), were found to decrease suicide attempts (Katz et al., 2013). Katz et al. (2013) suggest that no one program can be considered the "gold standard." Combining different aspects and pieces of programs may be necessary to maximize effectiveness. Similarly, Kong et al. (2016) reviewed current school-based intervention and prevention programming and found similar results (Bennett et al., 2015; Kong et al., 2016). Many literature reviews on suicide prevention have been conducted and all report similar findings in that current programming is lacking in rigor and fidelity (Bennett et al. 2015; Cusimano & Sameem, 2011; Katz et al., 2013; Kong et al., 2016). Current research should evaluate multiple components of effective programming (i.e., a "dosage effect"), treatment fidelity, and should utilize rigorous methodologies, like randomized controlled trials, all of which remain sparse in the current literature (Bennett et al., 2015; Breet et al., 2021; Brown et al., 2007).

A recent meta-analysis conducted by Breet et al. (2021) examining various suicide prevention programs across high schools and universities found promising results for differing outcomes (i.e., reducing non-fatal suicidal behavior, changing knowledge, attitudes, and stigma toward suicide and related topics, increasing help-seeking behavior); however, it also revealed the need for the expansion of research to develop a stronger evidence base to guide school-based suicide prevention efforts. In this meta-analysis, most of the studies included (71%) had sample sizes of less than 200 participants, failed to use randomized control trials, produced small to moderate effect sizes, and found differences in the effectiveness of standardized interventions implemented across settings (Breet et al., 2021).

Review of the literature indicates that programs are not utilizing appropriate measures of reliability and validity, are not implemented with fidelity, and results have not been replicated. Miller and Emanuele (2009) evaluated 13 studies regarding both universal and selected suicide intervention and prevention programs. Importantly, Miller and Emanuele (2009) revealed a mere 30% of studies utilized reliable and valid measures, only 20% of studies included fidelity of program implementation and not one study evaluated replicated effects. Similarly, Brann et al. (2021) performed a meta-analysis on 27 studies and concluded that high-quality studies are scarce in current literature. A major goal of suicide prevention and intervention programming is to reduce suicide attempts and suicide rates. Yet, research reveals that most programs excel in promoting suicide awareness and helping skills, but not for reduction of suicidal behavior (Brann et al., 2021).

There is also a lack of randomized control trials conducted on suicide prevention programming (Bennett et al., 2015; Brann et al., 2021;

Breet et al., 2021; Brown et al., 2007; Katz et al., 2013; Miller & Emanuele, 2009; Robinson et al., 2013). Efforts need to be made by researchers to address this existing gap in the literature to find evidence for effective programs and sufficient dosages. Gould et al. (2003) stressed the need for the field to develop empirically based programs for suicide prevention and intervention. Petersen (2019) criticized many programs for being the first of their kind and, in turn, lacking replication. Additionally, many programs rely on self-report solely to assess outcomes. Hence, the importance for programs to embed multi-method evaluation approaches in future research is critical.

A recent analysis of iatrogenic effects of evaluating suicidality using screening was conducted by DeCou and Schumann (2018). Importantly, they found there were no immediate, short-, or long-term impacts on individuals. Moreover, there was no significant rise in ideation. However, their analysis revealed that evaluating suicidality may impact mood negatively for some individuals (de Beurs et al., 2016; DeCou & Schumann, 2018). While these effects exist, it is important to note that these effects are not potent (DeCou & Schumann, 2018). Yet, Cukrowicz et al. (2010) indicate that these iatrogenic effects may exceed the positive impacts of suicide screening to individuals. Noteworthy studies were identified to yield positive effects on participants (Bailey et al., 2017; Cukrowicz et al., 2010; DeCou & Schumann, 2018; Eynan et al., 2014), while others note no significant iatrogenic effects (Bailey et al., 2017; Harris & Goh, 2017; Robinson et al., 2013). It will be important for future research to specifically determine if programs produce harmful effects for individuals.

Claim #8: Whole-School Programming Is the Best Approach

Although suicide is a significant and serious problem for youth in the United States, there has been limited evidence shown for whole-school programs targeting suicide prevention and intervention. One of the more prominent programs, the SOS, has demonstrated mixed findings. SOS is a universal, school-based prevention program designed for middle-school and high-school students (ages 11–17), with its goal to decrease suicide deaths and attempts by increasing student knowledge and adaptive attitudes about depression and encouraging help-seeking behaviors for themselves and for others. This program also aims to reduce the stigma of mental illness, acknowledge the importance of seeking help or treatment, as well as engaging parents and school professionals as partners in prevention through "gatekeeper" education, and encourage schools to cultivate community-based partnerships to support student mental health (Mindwise Innovations, n.d.; Suicide Prevention Resource Center, 2016).

Several studies evaluating SOS have found positive effects on increasing students' knowledge about depression and suicide (Aseltine & DeMartino, 2004; Aseltine et al., 2007; Schilling et al., 2016), more adaptive attitudes toward depression and suicide (Aseltine & DeMartino, 2004; Aseltine et al., 2007; Schilling et al., 2016), reduced suicidal attempts (Aseltine & DeMartino, 2004; Aseltine et al., 2007; Schilling et al., 2014, 2016), and reductions in suicide planning (Schilling et al., 2014, 2016). SOS has also been effective in screening for students who are at-risk for suicide at both the high-school and middle-school levels (e.g., Clark et al., 2022). However, there have been no significant effects on students' help-seeking behaviors (i.e., in the form of treatment, from a friend, or from an adult; Aseltine & DeMartino, 2004; Aseltine et al., 2007; Schilling et al., 2014), although the curriculum has been shown to increase student referral intentions for covert cues (i.e., warning signs that are more subtle or ambiguous, such as increased drug or alcohol use, social withdrawal) and keeping referral intentions for overt cues (i.e., talking about wanting to die, writing or expressing a goodbye message). Studies have also found that the SOS program had no significant impact on students' suicidal ideation (Aseltine & DeMartino, 2004; Aseltine et al., 2007; Schilling et al., 2016).

Although there have been emerging studies that follow students long-term after the implementation (e.g., Volungis, 2020), most of the evidence for the SOS program is for short-term effects (i.e., no outcomes reported beyond three months after the program). It is hard to determine the "dose" of interventions (e.g., quantity or intensity) needed to produce the intended response (e.g., clinical and/or statistical improvement; Robinson et al., 2019). For example, Ward-Ciesielski et al. (2017) found that a single session of dialectical-behavior therapy (DBT) did not reduce suicidal ideation, while other effective studies implemented a 20-week DBT intervention (e.g., Linehan et al., 2006; Mehlum et al., 2014), suggesting that longer-term therapy is needed.

Summary and Conclusion

There are many misconceptions in preventing suicide and effectively intervening when an individual is considering attempting suicide. Eight of these misconceptions have been reviewed in this chapter. What is most concerning for school administrators, teachers, and mental health professionals is that many programs that are marketed to schools have not been adequately nor rigorously researched. Suicide tends to be sensationalized in the popular press and simple, one-time programs are ineffective and in fact, might be damaging.

A comprehensive analysis of psychosocial treatments for suicide and self-injury urges researchers to advocate for randomized controlled trials, a rigorous examination of treatment mediators and moderators, and adapt and scale treatments in order to reach large numbers of youth (Glenn et al., 2019). Arguably, prevention and intervention programming that is coordinated and systematically delivered is the best approach to reach the greatest number of youth. Multi-Tiered System of Supports (MTSS; Cowan et al., 2013) is a widely recognized three-tiered framework used for a range of intervention service delivery models, offering more intensive interventions and more frequent progress monitoring at each tier. Utilizing this framework for suicide prevention recognizes the interconnected nature of social-emotional difficulties that can lead to suicidal thoughts and behaviors, as well as promoting school uniformity in responding and providing early intervention for students at-risk for suicide. MTSS indicates that approximately 80% of students need primary prevention strategies, 15% will need secondary prevention and intervention strategies, and 5% will need tertiary prevention and intervention strategies. In recent literature, there has been more focus on delivering prevention and intervention strategies embedded within an MTSS framework, including suicide prevention and intervention (Knoster et al., 2020; Schaffer, 2022; Singer et al., 2019).

Primary strategies (Tier 1) for suicide prevention should include those that aim to create a safe, supportive environment for all students and staff. Gatekeeper training, such as those included in the SOS program or QPR Gatekeeper training, and whole-school social-emotional learning, such as Committee for Children's Second Step Curriculum, situates themselves in primary prevention. Universal behavioral screenings (e.g., Behavior Intervention Monitoring System-2 (BIMAS-2); Devereux Student Strengths Assessment-mini (DSSA-mini) and teachings focused on mental wellness (e.g., Lifelines curriculum [Suicide Prevention Resource Center, 2007], SOS) also can be provided at a whole-school level to equip students with the knowledge of warning signs and how to seek help for themselves and their peers. Secondary supports embedded in Tier 2 aimed at students who may be at higher risk can include more specialized screenings assessing suicide risk (e.g., Columbia-Suicide Severity Rating Scale) and targeted small group interventions focusing on social skills (e.g., American Indian Life Skills curriculum; Suicide Prevention Resource Center, 2007). Creating support systems for students can include implementation of interventions to promote connection with school staff (e.g., Check and Connect). Safety planning with students found to be of lower risk can be situated in Tier 2 supports. Tertiary supports for prevention for students known to be at higher risk of suicide include individualized interventions and supports (e.g., school-based therapy based in cognitive-behavioral or dialectical behavioral therapy) and crisis response. Crisis response includes safety planning and brief suicide intervention plans, removal of access to lethal means, and referral and coordination with outside clinician or hospital for access to treatment and collaboration for re-entry plans.

Evidence-based suicide prevention and intervention programs are critical for addressing the alarming rates of youth suicide. Though many prevention and intervention programs exist and are marketed toward schools; their impact and effectiveness are questionable. Researchers have yet to answer the question, "what works under which conditions?" Promoting randomized controlled trials, using reliable and valid measures to assess outcomes, and research that examines treatment fidelity, dosage effects, and mental health treatment will help promote evidence-based programming for youth suicide.

References

Aseltine, R. H., & DeMartino, R. (2004). An outcome evaluation of the SOS suicide prevention program. *American Journal of Public Health*, *94*(3), 446–451. 10.2105/AJPH.94.3.446

Aseltine, R. H., James, A., Schilling, E. A., & Glanovsky, J. (2007). Evaluating the SOS suicide prevention program: A replication and extension. *BMC Public Health*, *7*(161). 10.1186/1471-2458-7-161

Bailey, E., Spittal, M. J., Pirkis, J., Gould, M., & Robinson, J. (2017). Universal suicide prevention in young people: An evaluation of the safeTALK program in Australian high schools. *Crisis: The Journal of Crisis Intervention and Suicide Prevention*, *38*(5), 300–308. 10.1027/0227-5910/a000465

Bennett, K., Rhodes, A. E., Duda, S., Cheung, A. H., Manassis, K., Links, P., Mushquash, C., Braunberger, P., Newton, A. S., Kutcher, S., Bridge, J. A., Santos, R. G., Manion, I. G., McLennan, J. D., Bagnell, A., Lipman, E., Rice, M., & Szatmari, P. (2015). A youth suicide prevention plan for Canada: A systematic review of reviews. *The Canadian Journal of Psychiatry/La Revue Canadienne de Psychiatrie*, *60*(6), 245–257. 10.1177/070674371506000603

Berman, A. L., Jobes, D. A., & Silverman, M. M. (2006). *Adolescent suicide: Assessment and intervention* (2nd ed.). Washington, DC: American Psychological Association. 10.1037/11285-000

Brann, K. L., Baker, D., Smith-Millman, M. K., Watt, S. J., & DiOrio, C. (2021). A meta- analysis of suicide prevention programs for school-aged youth. *Children and Youth Services Review*, *121*, 10.1016/j.childyouth.2020.105826

Breet, E., Matooane, M., Tomlinson, M., & Bantjes, J. (2021). Systematic review and narrative synthesis of suicide prevention in high-schools and universities: A research agenda for evidence-based practice. *BMC Public Health*, *21*, 1116, 1–21. 10.1186/s12889-021-11124-w

Brent, D., McMakin, D., Kennard, B., Goldstein, T., Mayes, T., & Douaihy, A. (2013). Protecting adolescents from self-harm: A critical review of intervention studies. *Journal of the American Academy of Child and Adolescent Psychiatry*, *52*(12), 1260–1271. 10.1016/j.jaac.2013.09.009

Bridge, J. A., Ruch, D. A., Sheftall, A. H., Hahm, H. C., O'Keefe, V. M., Fontanella, C. A., Brock, G., Campo, J. V., & Horowitz, L. M. (2023). Youth suicide during the first year of the COVID-19 pandemic. *Pediatrics*, *151*(3), 1–22. 10.1542/peds.2022-058375

Brown, C. H., Wyman, P. A., Brinales, J. M., & Gibbons, R. D. (2007). The role of randomized trials in testing interventions for the prevention of youth suicide. *International Review of Psychiatry*, *19*(6), 617–631. 10.1080/09540260701797779

Cai, H., Xie, X. M., Zhang, Q., Cui, X., Lin, J. X., Sim, K., Ungvari, G. S., Zhang, L., & Xiang, Y. T. (2021). Prevalence of suicidality in major depressive disorder: A systematic review and meta-analysis of comparative studies. *Frontiers in Psychiatry*, *12*, 690130. 10.3389/fpsyt.2021.690130

Callanan, V. J., & Davis, M. S., 2012. Gender differences in suicide methods. *Social Psychiatry and Psychiatric Epidemiology*. *47*, 857–869. 10.1007/s00127-011-0393-5

Centers for Disease Control (1988). CDC recommendations for a community plan for the prevention and containment of suicide clusters. *MMWR*, *37*(5–6), 1–12.

Centers for Disease Control and Prevention (2019). Youth risk behavior survey data. https://www.cdc.gov/healthyyouth/data/yrbs/index.htm

Cibis, A., Mergl, R., Bramesfeld, A., Althaus, D., Niklewski, G., Schmidtke, A., Hegerl, & U. (2012). Preference of lethal methods is not the only cause for higher suicide rates in males. *Journal of Affective Disorders*, *136*, 9–16. 10.101 6/j.jad.2011.08.03

Clark, K. N., Strissel, D., Malecki, C. K., Ogg, J., Demaray, M. K., & Eldridge, M. A., (2022). Evaluating the Signs of Suicide program: Middle school students at risk and staff acceptability. *School Psychology Review*, *51*(3), 354–369. 10. 1080/2372966X.2021.1936166

Cowan, K. C., Vaillancourt, K., Rossen, E., & Pollitt, K. (2013). *A framework for safe and successful schools [Brief]*. National Association of School Psychologists. http://www.nasponline.org/resources/handouts/Framework_for_Safe_and_ SuccessfulSchool_Environments.pdf

Cukrowicz, K., Smith, P., & Poindexter, E. (2010). The effect of participating in suicide research: Does participating in a research protocol on suicide and psychiatric symptoms increase suicide ideation and attempts? *Suicide and Life-Threatening Behavior*, *40*(6), 535–543. 10.1521/suli.2010.40.6.535

Cusimano, M. D., & Sameem, M. (2011). The effectiveness of middle and high school-based suicide prevention programmes for adolescents: A systematic review. *Injury Prevention*, *17*(1), 43–49. 10.1136/ip.2009.025502

Curtin S. C. (2020). State suicide rates among adolescents and young adults aged 10-24: United States, 2000-2018. *National vital statistics reports: from the Centers for Disease Control and Prevention, National Center for Health Statistics, National Vital Statistics System*, *69*(11), 1–10.

Daniel, S. S., & Goldston, D. B. (2009). Interventions for suicidal youth: A review of the literature and developmental considerations. *Suicide and Life-Threatening Behavior*, *39*(3), 252–268. 10.1521/suli.2009.39.3.252

de Beurs, D. P., Ghonech, R., Geraedts, A. S., & Kerkhof, A. J. F. M. (2016). Psychological distress because of asking about suicidal thoughts: A randomized controlled trial among students. *Archives of Suicide Research*, 20, 153–159. 10.1080/13811118.2015.1004475

DeCou, C. R., & Schumann, M. E. (2018). On the iatrogenic risk of assessing suicidality: A meta-analysis. *Suicide & Life-Threatening Behavior*, 48(5), 531–543. 10.1111/sltb.12368

Denning, D. G., Conwell, Y., King, D., & Cox, C. (2000). Method choice, intent, and gender in completed suicide. *Suicide and Life-Threatening Behavior*, 30(3), 282–288.

Eynan, R., Bergmans, Y., Antony, J., Cutcliffe, J. R., Harder, H. G., Ambreen, M., Balderson, K., & Links, P. S. (2014). Is research with suicidal participants risky business? In J. R. Cutcliffe, J. C. Santos, P. S. Links, J. Zaheer, H. G. Harder, F. Campbell, R. McCormick, K. Harder, Y. Bergmans, & R. Eynan (Eds.), *Routledge international handbook of clinical suicide research* (pp. 215–226). Routledge/Taylor & Francis Group.

Franklin, J. C., Ribeiro, J. D., Fox, K. R., Bentley, K. H., Kleiman, E. M., Huang, X., ... Nock, M. K. (2017). Risk factors for suicidal thoughts and behaviors: A meta-analysis of 50 years of research. *Psychological Bulletin*, 143, 187–232. 10.1037/bul0000084

Glenn, C. R., Esposito, E. C., Porter, A. C., & Robinson, D. J. (2019). Evidence base update of psychosocial treatments for self-injurious thoughts and behaviors in youth. *Journal of Clinical Child & Adolescent Psychology*, 48(3), 357–302. 10.1080/15374416.2019.1591281.

Glenn, C., Franklin, J., & Nock, M. (2015). Evidence-based psychosocial treatments for self-injurious thoughts and behaviors in youth. *Journal of Clinical Child & Adolescent Psychology*, 44(1), 1–29. 10.1080/15374416.2014.945211

Gould, M. S., & Davidson, L. (1988). Suicide contagion among adolescents. In A. R. Stiffman & R. A. Feldman (Eds.), *Advances in adolescent mental health* (pp. 29–59). Greenwich, CT: JAI Press.

Gould, M., Greenberg, T., Velting, D., & Shaffer, D. (2003). Youth suicide risk and preventive interventions: A review of the past 10 years. *Academy of Child and Adolescent Psychiatry*, 42(4), 386–405. 10.1097/01.CHI.0000046821.95464.CF

Gould, M., & Lake, A. M. (2013). *The contagion of suicide behavior: Impact of media reporting on suicide.* Forum on Global Violence Prevention: Based on Global Health Institute of Medicine, National Research Council: Washington DC: National Academies Press.

Harris, K. M., & Goh, M. T. (2017). Is suicide assessment harmful to participants? Findings from a randomized controlled trial. *International Journal of Mental Health Nursing*, 26(2), 181–190. 10.1111/inm.12223

Hill, R. M., & Pettit, J. W. (2019). Pilot randomized controlled trial of LEAP: A selective preventive intervention to reduce adolescents' perceived burdensomeness. *Journal of Clinical Child and Adolescent Psychology*, 48(sup1), S45–S56. 10.1080/15374416.2016.1188705

Kaess, M., Parzer, P., Haffner, J., Steen, R., Roos, J., Klett, M., Brunner, R., & Resch, F. (2011). Explaining gender differences in non-fatal suicidal behaviour among adolescents: A population-based study. *BMC Public Health*, 11(597) 1–7. 10.1186/1471-2458-11-597

Kalafat, J. (2003). School approaches to youth suicide prevention. *American Behavioral Scientist, 46*(9), 1211–1223. 10.1177/0002764202250665

Katz, C., Bolton, S. L., Katz, L. Y., Isaak, C., Tilston-Jones, T., & Sareen, J. (2013). A systematic review of school-based suicide prevention programs. *Depression and Anxiety, 30*(10), 1030–1045. 10.1002/da.22114

Knoster, T., Empson, D., & Perales, K. (2020). *PBIS Forum 2020: Applying the Multi-tiered Framework to Suicide Prevention. [Webinar]*. Center on Positive Behavioral Intervention Supports. https://www.pbis.org/video/session-a6-pbis-forum-2020-applying-the-multi-tiered-framework-to-suicide-prevention

Kong, L., Sareen, J., & Katz, L. Y. (2016). School-based suicide prevention programs. In *The international handbook of suicide prevention.* (pp. 725–742). Wiley. 10.1002/9781118903223.ch41

Kreski, N. T., Chen, Q., Olfson, M., Cerdá, M., Martins, S. S., Mauro, P. M., Hasin, D. S., & Keyes, K. M. (2022). National trends and disparities in bullying and suicidal behavior across demographic subgroups of US adolescents. *Journal of the American Academy of Child & Adolescent Psychiatry, 61*(12), 1435–1444. 10.1016/j.jaac.2022.04.011

Linehan, M. M., Comtois, K. A., Murray, A. M., Brown, M. Z., Gallop, R. J., Heard, H. L., Korslund, K. E., Tutek, D. A., Reynolds, S. K., & Lindenboim, N. (2006). Two-year randomized controlled trial and follow-up of dialectical behavior therapy vs therapy by experts for suicidal behaviors and borderline personality disorder. *Archives of General Psychiatry, 63*(7), 757–766. https://doi.org/archpsyc.63.7.757

Mazza, J. J. (1997). School-based suicide prevention programs: Are they effective?. *School Psychology Review, 26*(3), 382–396.

Mazza, J. J., & Reynolds, W. M. (2008). School-wide approaches to prevention of and treatment for depression and suicidal behaviors. In Doll, B. & Cummings, J. A. (Eds.), *Transforming school mental health services* (pp. 213–241). Thousand Oaks, CA: Corwin.

McKeown, R. E., Cuffe, S. P., & Schulz, R. M. (2006). US suicide rates by age group, 1970–2002: An examination of recent trends. *American Journal of Public Health, 96*(10), 1744–1751. 10.2105/AJPH.2005.066951

Mehlum, L., Tømoen, A. J., Ramberg, M., Haga, E., Diep, L. M., Laberg, S., Larsson, B. S., Stanley, B. H., Miller, A. L., Sund, A. M., & Grøholt, B. (2014). Dialectical behavior therapy for adolescents with repeated suicidal and self-harming behavior: A randomized trial. *Journal of the American Academy of Child and Adolescent Psychiatry, 53*(10), 1082–1091. 10.1016/j.jaac.2014.07.003

Miller, D. N., & DuPaul, G. J. (1996). School-based prevention of adolescent suicide: Issues, obstacles, and recommendations for practice. *Journal of Emotional and Behavioral Disorders, 4*(4), 221–230. 10.1177/106342669600400403

Miller, A. L., & Emanuele, J. M. (2009). Children and adolescents at risk of suicide. In P. M. Kleespies (Ed.), *Behavioral emergencies: An evidence-based resource for evaluating and managing risk of suicide, violence, and victimization* (pp. 79–101). American Psychological Association. 10.1037/11865-004

MindWise Innovations(n.d.). *Suicide prevention programs overview.* https://www.mindwise.org/what-we-offer/suicide-prevention-programs/

Moskos, M. A., Achilles, J., & Gray, D. (2004). Adolescent suicide myths in the United States. *Crisis: The Journal of Crisis Intervention and Suicide Prevention*, 25(4), 176–182. 10.1027/0227-5910.25.4.176

Pérez Barrero, S. A., & Sereno Batista, A. (2001) Conocimientos de un grupo de adolescentes sobre la conducta suicida. *Revista Internacional de Tanatología y Suicidio*, 1(2), 7–10.

Pérez Barrero, S. A. (2003). *Psicoterapia para aprender a vivir*. Editorial Oriente.

Petersen, P. M. (2019). Suicide prevention in schools. *Intuition: The BYU Undergraduate Journal of Psychology*, 14(1), 10. https://scholarsarchive.byu.edu/intuition/vol14/iss1/10

QPR Institute. (2011). *QPR for Schools*. https://qprinstitute.com/

Reynolds, W. M. (1988). *Suicidal ideation questionnaire: Professional manual*. Odessa, FL: Psychological Assessment Resources.

Reynolds, W. M., & Mazza, J. J. (1994). Suicide and suicidal behaviors in children and adolescents. In W. M. Reynolds & H. F. Johnston (Eds.), *Handbook of depression in children and adolescents* (pp. 525–580). Plenum Press. 10.1007/978-1-4899-1510-8_24

Robinson, J., Cox, G., Malone, A., Williamson, M., Baldwin, G., Fletcher, K., & O'Brien, M. (2013). A systematic review of school-based interventions aimed at preventing, treating, and responding to suicide-related behavior in young people. *Crisis: The Journal of Crisis Intervention and Suicide Prevention*, 34(3), 164–182. 10.1027/0227-5910/a000168

Robinson, L., Delgadillo, J., & Kellett, S. (2019). The dose-response effect in routinely delivered psychological therapies: A systematic review. *Psychotherapy Research*, 30(1), 79–96. 10.1080/10503307.2019.1566676

Rowe, S. L., French, R. S., Henderson, C., Ougrin, D., Slade, M., & Moran, P. (2014). Help-seeking behaviour and adolescent self-harm: A systematic review. *The Australian and New Zealand Journal of Psychiatry*, 48(12), 1083–1095. 10.1177/0004867414555718

Schaffer, G. E. (2022). Chapter 6: Suicide prevention and intervention. In *Multi-tiered systems of support: A practice guide to implementing preventative practice* (pp. 107–136). Los Angeles, CA: SAGE Publications, Inc.

Schilling, E. A., Lawless, M., Buchanan, L., & Aseltine, R. H. (2014). "Signs of Suicide" shows promise as a middle school suicide prevention program. *Suicide and Life-Threatening Behavior*, 44(6), 653–667. 10.1111/sltb.12097

Schilling, E. A., Aseltine, R. H., & James., A. (2016). The SOS suicide prevention program: Further evidence of efficacy and effectiveness. *Prevention Science*, 17, 157–166. 10.1007/s11121-015-0594-3

Schmutte, T. J., & Wilkinson, S. T. (2020). Suicide in older adults with and without known mental illness: Results from the national violent death reporting system, 2003–2016. *American Journal of Preventive Medicine*, 58(4), 584–590.

Simes, D., Shochet, I., Murray, K., & Sands, I. G. (2022). A systematic review of qualitative research of the experiences of young people and their caregivers affected by suicidality and self-harm: implications for family-based treatment. *Adolescent Research Review*, 7(2), 211–233.

Singer, J. B., Erbacher, T. A., & Rosen, P. (2019). School-based suicide prevention: A framework for evidence-based practice. *School Mental Health*, *11*, 54–71. 10.1007/s12310-018-9245-8

Slovak, K., & Singer, J. B. (2012). Engaging parents of suicidal youth in a rural environment. *Child & Family Social Work*, *17*, 212–221. https://doi.org/10.1111/j.13652206.2012.00826.x

Suicide Prevention Resource Center (2007). *American Indian Life Skills*. https://sprc.org/online-library/american-indian-life-skills-developmentzuni-life-skills-development

Suicide Prevention Resource Center (2016). *SOS signs of suicide middle school and high school prevention programs*. https://sprc.org/online-library/sos-signs-suicide

Värnik, A., Kõlves, K., van der Feltz-Cornelis, C. M., Marusi, A., Oskarsson, H., Palmer, A., Reisch, T., Scheerder, G., Arensman, E., Aromaa, E., Giupponi, G., Gusmäo, R., Maxwell, M., Pull, C., Szekely, A., Sola, V. P., & Hegerl, U. (2008). Suicide methods in Europe: A gender-specific analysis of countries participating in the "European Alliance against Depression." *Journal of Epidemiology and Community Health*, *62*(6), 545–551. 10.1136/jech.2007.065391

Volungis, A. M. (2020). The signs of suicide (SOS) prevention program pilot study: High school implementation recommendations. *North American Journal of Psychology*, *22*(3), 455–468. https://digitalcommons.assumption.edu/psychology-faculty/21

Ward-Ciesielski, E. F., Tidik, J. A., Edwards, A. J., & Linehan, M. M. (2017). Comparing brief interventions for suicidal individuals not engaged in treatment: A randomized clinical trial. *Journal of Affective Disorders*, *222*, 153–161. 10.1016/j.jad.2017.07.011

Weissman, M. M., Bland, R. C., Canino, G. J., Greenwald, S., Hwu, H.-G., Joyce, P. R., Karam, E. G., Lee, C.-K., Lellouch, J., Lepine, J.-P., Newman, S. C., Rubio-Stipec, M., Wells, J. E., Wickramaratne, P. J., Wittchen, H.-U., & Yeh, E.-K. (1999). Prevalence of suicide ideation and suicide attempts in nine countries. *Psychological Medicine*, *29*(1), 9–17. 10.1017/S0033291798007867

World Health Organization (2019). *Suicide in the world: Global health estimates*. Geneva: World Health Organization; 2018. Licence: CC BY-NC-SA 3.0 IGO. https://apps.who.int/iris/bitstream/handle/10665/274603/9789241565639-eng.pdf

Wu, P., Katic, B., Liu, X., Fan, B., & Fuller, C. (2010). Mental health service use among suicidal adolescents: Findings from a US National Community Survey. *Psychiatric Services*, *61*(1), 17–24. 10.1176/appi.ps.61.1.17

Zenere, F. J. (2009). Recognizing and addressing suicide contagion are essential to successful suicide postvention efforts. *Principal Leadership*, *10*, 12–16. Retrieved from http://www.nasponline.org/resources/principals/Suicide_Clusters_NASSP_Sept_%2009.pdf.

Zenere, F. J., III, & Lazarus, P. J. (1997). The decline of youth suicidal behavior in an urban, multicultural public school system following the introduction of a suicide prevention and intervention program. *Suicide and Life-Threatening Behavior*, *27*, 387–403.

5 Prevention Programs for Risky Behavior

Marisa E. Marraccini, Lauren E. Delgaty, and Telieha J. Middleton

Risk behaviors occurring during childhood and adolescence may include but are not limited to, alcohol and substance use, tobacco use, driving while intoxicated, failing to wear a seat belt, and risky sex behaviors, including unprotected sexual intercourse. The Youth Risk Surveillance System (YRBSS), which measures how trends in risk behaviors may change over time, was developed in the late 1980s to address the leading causes of mortality and morbidity among children and adolescents and adapted for use in schools in the 1990s (Kolbe et al., 1993). The most recent YRBSS addresses behaviors across six health-related behaviors contributing to leading causes of death and disability in youth and young adults: behaviors contributing to unintentional injuries and violence; sexual behaviors that may contribute to sexually transmitted infections (STIs) and unintended pregnancies; alcohol and other drug use; tobacco use; dietary behaviors considered to be unhealthy; and inadequate physical inactivity (YRBSS Overview | YRBSS | Adolescent and School Health | CDC, 2020). Despite a higher prevalence of risk behaviors among adolescents compared to children and adults (de Guzman & Bosch, 2007; Somerville & Casey, 2010; Substance Abuse and Mental Health Services Administration (US) & Office of the Surgeon General (US), 2016), the past few decades are marked by a decline in alcohol and most drug use among youth (Miech et al., 2021), and a trend toward increased contraception use during sexual activity (Lindberg et al., 2021).

School-based drug prevention programs have been delivered since the 1960s, with an uptick considering the landmark Anti-Drug Abuse Acts of 1986 and 1988 (Gorman, 1998). Additionally, efforts to prevent the spread of sexually transmitted infections (STIs; then termed "venereal disease") led to the adoption of sex education programs even earlier, during the beginning of the 1900s (Imber, 1982). Historically, school-based prevention programs have involved: (1) information dissemination; (2) affective approaches, such as clarification of values and decision-making; and (3) social skills and beliefs (Flay & Collins, 2005). This

DOI: 10.4324/9781003266181-7

evolution marks a shift from passive approaches aimed at changing knowledge, toward more dynamic approaches that integrate communication and social learning theories that focus on changing behaviors (Flay & Collins, 2005). While psychoeducation related to risks associated with sex and drug use remains prominent, multi-component school-based programs to enhance refusal skills have consistently demonstrated small effects for substance use (Hale et al., 2014).

Given the relevancy of school social interactions for influencing risk behaviors, numerous policy makers and researchers have called upon schools to continue to deliver prevention programs addressing risky sexual behaviors, drugs, and alcohol (Goldfarb & Lieberman, 2020; Hale et al., 2014). Some of the most prominent examples of prevention programs related to substance use include Drug Abuse Resistance Education (DARE) and Fatal Vision Goggles, and prominent examples of prevention programs related to sexual activity include abstinence-only prevention programs and infant simulator dolls. In this chapter, we will critically examine all four of these programs.

Examining the Claims

Drug Abuse Resistance Education (DARE)

One of the most widely disseminated programs initially implemented without a compelling scientific evidence base is the popular anti-drug education program, DARE. The program was founded through an effort by the Los Angeles Police Department and the Los Angeles United County School District in 1983 (Caputi & McLellan, 2017; Ennett, Rosenbaum, et al., 1994). Upon its conception, DARE aspired to combat drug use and gang violence in the Los Angeles area through instruction with a uniformed police officer (Caputi & McLellan, 2017). DARE includes courses for elementary, middle school, and high school students with a core curriculum for elementary school students aimed at fifth and sixth graders (Ennett, Rosenbaum, et al., 1994; Rosenbaum, 2007).

Despite a significant lack of evidence, DARE's core curriculum was rapidly implemented across the United States, and throughout the late 1990s, DARE was administered in approximately 70% of U.S. school districts (Rosenbaum & Hanson, 1998). Six million students were reported to participate in DARE during the 1993 school year (Hansen & McNeal, 1997). A sizeable amount of federal funding and a rigorous marketing campaign continued to support the circulation of DARE (Hansen & McNeal, 1997; West & O'Neal, 2004). Yet, DARE's effectiveness was long questioned by researchers in peer-reviewed scientific journals (Birkeland et al., 2005; Vincus et al., 2010). Although findings have demonstrated that DARE may have some positive, immediate effects on student outcomes, including self-perceived increases in social skills and assertiveness, increased positivity in attitudes toward police, and less favorable views on drugs (Birkeland et al., 2005; Harmon, 1993; Lynam et al., 1999; Ringwalt et al., 1991; Rosenbaum, 2007), these immediate effects did not address the primary goal of DARE – prevention of drug use.

Nonetheless, studies exploring the short-term effects of drug use behaviors following participation in the program have generally revealed negligible impacts on drug use with small effect sizes (Birkeland et al., 2005; Harmon, 1993; Vincus et al., 2010; West & O'Neal, 2004). When psychosocial effects and reduction in drug use were found to exist, the improvements typically dissipated within one to two years following program completion (Clayton et al., 1996; Dukes et al., 1996; Ennett, Rosenbaum, et al., 1994; Rosenbaum & Hanson, 1998). One study, commonly cited in the media, even found a small, but significant *increase* in drug use within a group of suburban students following the completion of the program (Rosenbaum & Hanson, 1998). Longitudinal data have also demonstrated little to no impact on drug use following completion of the program (Clayton et al., 1996; Dukes et al., 1996; Ennett, Rosenbaum, et al., 1994; Lynam et al., 1999; Rosenbaum & Hanson, 1998).

The DARE curriculum attempts to reduce substance use by addressing psychological processes that are thought to be mediators for drug use (Hansen & McNeal, 1997), including teaching children how to resist peer pressure (Ringwalt et al., 1991). Researchers have postulated that the program's failure may be due to the DARE curriculum having minimal to no effects on these mediators (Hansen & McNeal, 1997; Rosenbaum & Hanson, 1998). Researchers have also suggested a weak association between the hypothesized mediators and substance use, meaning that any program that targets these variables would be unable to create measurable change (Hansen & McNeal, 1997).

Despite these findings, DARE continued to persist in public schools (Clayton et al., 1996). Lynam et al. (1999) provide possible reasons for this persistence. First, its popularity may have stemmed from its intuitive nature – that is, teaching children about avoiding drug use and other risk behaviors seemed like a logical solution. Moreover, adults may have attributed behaviors among adolescents who did not engage in drug experimentation to the program's success, in part because they may have believed (or were led to believe) that drug use was far more prevalent among adolescents than it actually was. In turn, such ongoing public support may have distracted policy makers and researchers from considering critical examination of the program's effectiveness.

Even some of the professionals aware of the research demonstrating the negligible effects of DARE chose to implement the program. Relatedly, Birkeland et al. (2005) make several points. First, administrators described maintaining the program to improve the relationships between students and police officers. Second, educators also stated that they felt researchers "missed the mark" when looking for substantial reductions in drug use as the success measure for DARE. Finally, instead, the educators may have placed their positive personal experiences with the program above empirical evidence and chose to continue including it in their curriculum.

In the early 2000s, DARE responded to the growing criticisms stemming from a robust literature base demonstrating its negligible effects. The organization changed leadership and began developing and testing a new curriculum (Caputi & McLellan, 2017) based on strengthening decision-making skills and protective factors that have been demonstrated to increase resiliency in at-risk youth (Singh et al., 2011). DARE later partnered with the *Keepin' it REAL* program, a culturally sensitive program created by Pennsylvania State University, and continued to undergo several curriculum revisions in an attempt to improve the program's effectiveness (Caputi & McLellan, 2017).

Despite its promise, evaluations of the new DARE version of the *Keepin' it REAL* (Refuse, Explain, Avoid, Leave) program have demonstrated mixed results for reducing substance use (Jewell et al., 2018). Researchers have expressed concern that nationwide implementation of DARE's *Keepin' it REAL* continues without rigorous, peer-reviewed evaluations of the program's effectiveness for drug prevention among the students receiving the intervention (Caputi & McLellan, 2017; Jewell et al., 2018). Note, however, that the co-creators of the *Keepin' it REAL* program have questioned such critique, reporting that these critical analyses included incorrect versions of the program and mis-attributed program development as targeting Hispanic youth only (as opposed to culturally diverse youth; Miller-Day & Hecht, 2017). A recent, independent evaluation of the program suggested a significant reduction of alcohol and drug use 4 months following the intervention (University of North Carolina at Greensboro, 2022); however, the long-term effects of the intervention remain unknown.

Fatal Vision Goggles

Fatal Vision Goggles facilitate an experience that simulates visual impairments similar to those from alcohol, allowing users to experience visual distortions across varying levels of alcohol consumption (e.g., from blood alcohol content of .06 to above .10; Hawkins & Vraga, 2018). The goggles facilitate visual field shifts and disturbances to equilibrium, resulting in impaired balance, vision, reaction time, and judgment (*Fatal Vision® Polydrug [Alcohol & Marijuana] Goggles – Program Kit*, n.d.). Note, however, that without additional cognitive demands, the effects of Fatal Vision Goggles are limited to visual impairments and do not mimic cognitive impairments associated with alcohol (Irwin et al., 2019). Since their development in 1996, several iterations have been produced, including Fatal Vision Polydrug Goggles [Alcohol & Marijuana] and Fatal Vision Marijuana Goggles (*Fatal Vision® Polydrug [Alcohol & Marijuana] Goggles – Program Kit*, n.d.).

Fatal Vision Goggles have been used as a component of several drug and alcohol prevention programs (including some DARE programs; Jewell et al., 2004), as well as driver education programs (McCartney et al., 2017). According to a 1997 Innocorp newsletter, Fatal Vision Goggles were adopted by schools, as well as other agencies (e.g., law enforcement, universities), across the United States and internationally (Jewell et al., 2004). Although the developers reported the activity to be evidence-based, schools and other institutions widely adopted their use prior to any rigorous empirical evidence.

Although several studies suggest short-term changes in college students' attitudes and/or intentions toward drinking and driving (Hennessy et al., 2006; Jewell et al., 2004; J. Jewell & Hupp, 2005), with effects most potent among those already engaging in alcohol use (Hawkins & Vraga, 2018; Hennessy et al., 2006), effects do not appear to translate to meaningful changes in behavior (Jewell & Hupp, 2005). That is, the use of Fatal Vision Goggles as a prevention strategy has not been found to lead to reductions in drinking and driving in college students (Jewell & Hupp, 2005; Meeker & Kehl, 2020) or explored as a preventative strategy in most other populations. Moreover, studying the use of Fatal Vision Goggles with middle school students, Morales and Day (2017) found no significant changes in attitudes toward drinking and driving, perhaps because middle schoolers have no driving experience (making it difficult for them to grasp the seriousness of the consequences involved). Although the use of Fatal Vision Goggles may have utility for mimicking some alcohol-related impairments in order help youth better understand the effects of alcohol on driving performance (McCartney et al., 2017), research to date does not support their use as a component of programs aimed at preventing drinking and driving.

Nonetheless, Fatal Vision Goggles are still promoted as a component for programs aimed at preventing drinking and driving behaviors. For example, they are promoted and sold by educator and teacher aid programs (Nasco Education, 2022) and preventative programs marketed to and adopted by schools (e.g., Reduce Teen Crashes [*Fatal Vision Goggles*, 2022]), Champions for a Drug Free Muhlenberg County [*"Fatal Vision Goggles" Show Teens the Dangers of DUI*, n.d.]). They have also been integrated into annual college prevention programs (e.g., University of Minnesota Morris [Jrray, 2016]). Moreover, Fatal Vision Goggle activities are provided as a component of transportation safety programs and drug and alcohol prevention programs across the country (e.g., the Mississippi Department of Transportation's safety programs (*Goggles—MS Safety Education*, n.d.), New Hampshire's Liquor Commission Division of Enforcement (*Fatal Choices | Education and Training | NH Liquor Commission, Division of Enforcement*, n.d.), Maryland-National Capital Park and Planning Commission (*Fatal Vision Program | MNCPPC, MD*, n.d.) and Zero Deaths Maryland (*Fatal Vision Goggles*, n.d.).

Abstinence-Only Sex Education

Abstinence-only sex education programs teach school-aged youth about the benefits of abstaining from sex until marriage, such as preventing STIs and accidental pregnancies (Santelli et al., 2006). This approach is based on the idea that preventing youth from engaging in sexual behaviors *completely* will reduce the risk for all negative outcomes associated with sex. This approach is also based on the assumption of innocence in childhood, chastity, and the morality surrounding sexual activity outside of marriage (Fields, 2005; Gilbert, 2010). Accordingly, abstinence-only programs do not use other STI and pregnancy prevention practices such as teaching about condom use and other forms of contraception (Kirby, 2008). Historically, these programs have been supported by the federal government (Santelli et al., 2006), despite evidence that they are ineffective for preventing sexual activity or reducing risk for pregnancy and STIs (Kohler et al., 2008) and the public belief that abstinence-only sex education programs by themselves do not prevent unplanned pregnancies (Bleakley et al., 2006). As Santelli et al. (2006) stated, abstinence-only programs persist due to "an artful mix of science and pseudoscience" (p. 839).

Unfortunately, abstinence-only curriculums may exaggerate the negative or adverse outcomes from sexual activity and also present false or distorted information related to reproductive health (Santelli et al., 2006). Although findings from one study support long-term gains in knowledge, as well as increases in intent to remain abstinent among elementary, middle, and high school students (Denny & Young, 2006), most research indicates that abstinence-only programs have negligible effects on abstinence, STIs, and unintended pregnancies (Heels, 2019; Kirby, 2008; Lindberg & Maddow-Zimet, 2012). Moreover, because abstinence-only programs are based on heteronormative practices (e.g., they focus exclusively on heterosexual relationships), they can have harmful effects for youth identifying as lesbian, gay, bisexual, transgender, questioning, intersex, two-spirit, and queer (LGBTQ+; Heels, 2019; Santelli et al., 2006). Youth identifying under the LGBTQ+ umbrella already face numerous obstacles in accessing healthcare (Aleshire et al., 2019), intensifying the negative effects of abstinence-only practices.

In contrast to abstinence-only sex education, comprehensive sex education programs are supported by a substantial body of literature (Goldfarb & Lieberman, 2020). Although comprehensive sex education commonly includes information about abstinence in the curriculum, it also focuses on other aspects of sex education such as information on contraceptives, practicing safe sex, and sexuality (Leung et al., 2019). Several studies and reviews have reported on the benefits proffered by comprehensive sex education programs that are not found in abstinence-only programs (Kirby, 2008; Kohler et al., 2008).

In an exploration of national adolescent pregnancy and birthrate data from 2005, Stanger-Hall and Hall (2011) found that sex education laws and policies emphasizing abstinence-only approaches were associated with increased rates of teen pregnancies and birth. Nonetheless, findings from a content analysis of state statutes, state board of education policies, and state department of education or public instruction curriculum standards indicate that most state policies (approximately three-quarters) continue to prioritize abstinence, without additional requirements regarding contraceptive methods to prevent risk (Hall et al., 2019).

Infant Simulator Dolls

Infant simulator dolls are designed to mimic the demands of child-rearing in real life. For example, *Baby Think It Over* includes a computerized infant simulator program that can be incorporated within other curriculums (Hoyt & Broom, 2002). The program has been adapted for use across the world (e.g., *Virtual Infant Parenting (VIP) Programme* in Western Australia; Brinkman et al., 2016). In its original conception, participants received infant simulator dolls that were designed to cry every 45 minutes to 6 hours, with variable settings to replicate "difficult" or "colicky" infants to those considered "easy" (Strachan & Gorey, 1997). This approach is based on the premise that facilitating realistic appraisal of future consequences and rewards in adolescents will support their subsequent decisions such as delaying sexual activity (Strachan & Gorey, 1997).

In their initial quasi-experimental study, Strachan and Gorey (1997) provided infant simulator dolls to six adolescents, considering an additional 17 vicariously exposed to the intervention because they were in the same class. Although not statistically significant, the researchers reported improved understanding of realistic parenting based on trend-level findings, extrapolating significance and large effects based on estimates of a *hypothetical* doubled sample size demonstrating the same changes (note that such a generalization from a small sample size toward population effects is significantly flawed, considering findings may be due to chance and high degrees of error; Tipton et al., 2017). Nonetheless, following this pilot study, by 2001 the intervention *Baby Think it Over* was described by the manufacturer to have been used with more than 1 million students, adopted across all 50 states of the United States and across the globe, and integrated into school systems (Somers & Fahlman, 2001).

Some of the early pilot studies continuing to explore the effects of these approaches boasted improvements in perceptions and intentions related to childcare and pregnancy, such as the challenges of childcare (e.g., the time and effort involved in caregiving) and the consequences of sex (de Anda, 2006; Didion & Gatzke, 2004; Divine & Cobbs, 2001; Out & Lafreniere, 2001), as well as reinforcing plans to delay planned pregnancies (Borr, 2009). Yet, studies examining outcomes related to knowledge and attitudes about sex and sexual or contraceptive behavior did not support significant effects of infant simulator dolls (Barnett, 2006; Somers & Fahlman, 2001), with more rigorous studies failing to replicate effects for attitude changes about teen pregnancy and parenting (Herrman et al., 2011; Out & Lafreniere, 2001; Somers & Fahlman, 2001). In a study conducted with 109 girls in middle school, the more difficult the simulated experience felt, the more students endorsed believing that caring for a real infant would be easier, with no significant effects on intentions to become teen parents from pre to post-intervention (although the researchers found a slight increase, from 12% to 15%, results were not significant; Kralewski & Stevens-Simon, 2000). In a study exploring teacher, parent, and student perspectives on the intervention, Tingle (2002) reported that although both teachers and parents reported favorable outcomes, minimal effects related to perspectives and attitudes on parenting among students were supported.

Despite limited evidence, as recently as 2016, Realityworks (the manufacturer) reported that infant simulator dolls were being used in school- and community-based adolescent prevention programs across 89 countries, including 67% of US school districts (Brinkman et al., 2016). However, findings from the first randomized control trial addressing infant simulator dolls (part of the *VIP Programme*) conducted in Australia put these practices into question (Brinkman et al., 2016). In their study, a total of 57 schools were randomized into treatment (*VIP*) and control (standard health education curriculum) conditions, including a total of 2,834 girls aged 13–15 years participating in the program between 2003 and 2006. An analysis of childbirths and induced abortions by the age of 20 indicated negligible effects overall, with those receiving the infant simulator doll demonstrating a higher overall pregnancy risk compared to those receiving standard health education curriculums. Yet, as recently as 2019, *The New York Times* estimated that infant simulator dolls were used by two-thirds of US school districts, with one school reporting that their reasoning for the program was not for pregnancy prevention, but rather, for understanding the challenges of parenting. The principal of the school was quoted as saying, "While we do not have research to support the statistical effect of this project, we do have decades of written reports by our students which speak eloquently to the perspectives they have gained" (Leeland, 2019, p. 8). This quote illustrates the problem of anecdotes being prioritized over rigorous research designs.

Summary and Conclusion

A common theme across pseudoscientific approaches to risky behavior prevention is the values and convictions held by interventionists and policy makers that reinforce resistance to evidence conflicting with these beliefs. Federal funding for abstinence-only education required that schools teach about the harmful effects of consensual sex outside of marriage, despite no research to substantiate such a lesson (Santelli et al., 2006). A 2017 article about the history of DARE published in *The Washington Post* (Ingraham, 2017) describes a 1994 *Herald-Journal* news article (Marlow & Rhodes, 1994) showcasing the Justice Department and executive DARE's criticism and disbelief at the early research (Ennett, Tobler, et al., 1994) refuting the effectiveness of the program. According to the article, the Justice Department refused to publish the findings, criticizing the rigor of the study (despite its acceptance following rigorous peer review to the *American Journal of Public Health*). The Executive Director of DARE was also quoted as saying, "I don't get it. It's like kicking Santa Claus to me ... We're as pure as the driven snow" (Marlow & Rhodes, 1994, A3). Likewise, executives of Realitywork (the manufacturer of *Baby Think It Over*) remain critical of Brinkman et al.' (2016) landmark findings that pointed to the negative effects of infant simulator dolls, explaining in *the New York Times* that the findings do not apply to their specific curriculum (Leeland, 2019).

Thus, the need to critically examine and question dominant risk behavior prevention programs remains, requiring us to question: *What risk behavior prevention practices are we currently using that lack empirical evidence today? What tradition-based practices have we inherited that were developed in the context of exclusionary and oppressive practices to underrepresented groups?* Although school psychologists may face difficulty in tackling programs born out of policy and practices informed by public and federal beliefs and values, they are uniquely positioned to pose and address these questions.

References

Aleshire, M. E., Ashford, K., Fallin-Bennett, A., & Hatcher, J. (2019). Primary care providers' attitudes related to LGBTQ people: A narrative literature review. *Health Promotion Practice*, 20(2), 173–187. 10.1177/1524839918778835

Barnett, J. E. (2006). Evaluating "baby think it over" infant simulators: A comparison group study. *Adolescence, 41*(161), 103–111.

Birkeland, S., Murphy-Graham, E., & Weiss, C. (2005). Good reasons for ignoring good evaluation: The case of the drug abuse resistance education (D.A.R.E.) program. *Evaluation and Program Planning, 28*(3), 247–256. 10.1016/j.evalprogplan.2005.04.001

Bleakley, A., Hennessy, M., & Fishbein, M. (2006). Public opinion on sex education in US schools. *Archives of Pediatrics & Adolescent Medicine, 160*(11), 1151–1156. 10.1001/archpedi.160.11.1151

Borr, M. L. (2009). Baby think it over: A weekend with an infant simulator. *Journal of Family & Consumer Sciences Education. 27*(2), 11.

Brinkman, S. A., Johnson, S. E., Codde, J. P., Hart, M. B., Straton, J. A., Mittinty, M. N., & Silburn, S. R. (2016). Efficacy of infant simulator programmes to prevent teenage pregnancy: A school-based cluster randomised controlled trial in Western Australia. *The Lancet, 388*(10057), 2264–2271. 10.1016/S0140-6736(16)30384-1

Caputi, T. L., & McLellan, A. T. (2017). Truth and D.A.R.E.: Is D.A.R.E.'s new Keepin' it REAL curriculum suitable for American nationwide implementation?. *Drugs: Education, Prevention and Policy, 24*(1), 49–57. 10.1080/09687637. 2016.1208731

Clayton, R. R., Cattarello, A. M., & Johnstone, B. M. (1996). The effectiveness of drug abuse resistance education (Project DARE): 5-year follow-up results. *Preventive Medicine, 25*(3), 307–318. 10.1006/pmed.1996.0061

de Anda, D. (2006). Baby think it over: Evaluation of an infant simulation intervention for adolescent pregnancy prevention. *Health & Social Work, 31*(1), 26–35. 10.1093/hsw/31.1.26

de Guzman, M. R., & Bosch, K. (2007). G07-1715 high-risk behaviors among youth. *Historical Materials from University of Nebraska-Lincoln Extension.* https://digitalcommons.unl.edu/extensionhist/4099

Denny, G., & Young, M. (2006). An evaluation of an abstinence-only sex education curriculum: An 18-month follow-up. *Journal of School Health, 76*(8), 414–422. 10.1111/j.1746-1561.2006.00135.x

Didion, J., & Gatzke, H. (2004). The baby think It Over™ experience to prevent teen pregnancy: A postintervention evaluation. *Public Health Nursing, 21*(4), 331–337. 10.1111/j.0737-1209.2004.21406.x

Divine, J. H., & Cobbs, G. (2001). The effects of infant simulators on early adolescents. *Adolescence, 36*(143), 593–600.

Dukes, R. L., Ullman, J. B., & Stein, J. A. (1996). Three-year follow-up of drug abuse resistance education (D.A.R.E.). *Evaluation Review, 20*(1), 49–66. 10. 1177/0193841X9602000103

Ennett, S. T., Rosenbaum, D. P., Flewelling, R. L., Bieler, G. S., Ringwalt, C. L., & Bailey, S. L. (1994). Long-term evaluation of drug abuse resistance education. *Addictive Behaviors, 19*(2), 113–125. 10.1016/0306-4603(94)90036-1

Ennett, S. T., Tobler, N. S., Ringwalt, C. L., & Flewelling, R. L. (1994). How effective is drug abuse resistance education? A meta-analysis of Project DARE outcome evaluations. *American Journal of Public Health, 84*(9), 1394–1401. 10.2105/AJPH.84.9.1394

Fatal Choices | Education and Training | NH Liquor Commission, Division of Enforcement. (n.d.). Retrieved November 11, 2022, from https://www.nh.gov/liquor/enforcement/education/fatal-choices.htm

Fatal Vision® Polydrug [Alcohol & Marijuana] Goggles—Program Kit. (n.d.). Innocorp Ltd. Retrieved November 11, 2022, from https://www.fatalvision.com/product/fatal-vision-alcohol-marijuana-combo-program-kit/

Fatal Vision Goggles. (n.d.). Zero Deaths Maryland & Vision Zero - Maryland Highway Safety Office. Retrieved November 11, 2022, from https://zerodeathsmd.gov/resources/community-outreach/fatal-vision-goggles/

Fatal Vision Goggles. (2022, April 26). Reduce OH Crashes. https://www.reduceohcrashes.com/activities/fatal-vision-goggles

"Fatal Vision Goggles" show teens the dangers of DUI. (n.d.). Retrieved November 11, 2022, from https://www.tristatehomepage.com/news/local-news/muhlenberg-county/fatal-vision-goggles-show-teens-the-dangers-of-dui/

Fatal Vision Program | MNCPPC, MD. (n.d.). Retrieved November 11, 2022, from https://www.mncppc.org/2762/Fatal-Vision-Program

Fields, J. (2005). "Children having children": Race, innocence, and sexuality education. *Social Problems*, 52(4), 549–571.

Flay, B. R., & Collins, L. M. (2005). Historical review of school-based randomized trials for evaluating problem behavior prevention programs. *The Annals of the American Academy of Political and Social Science*, 599(1), 115–146.

Gilbert, J. (2010). Ambivalence only? Sex education in the age of abstinence. *Sex Education*, 10(3), 233–237.

Goggles—MS Safety Education. (n.d.). Retrieved November 11, 2022, from https://mdot.ms.gov/safetyeducation/programs/survive-your-drive/goggles.aspx

Goldfarb, E. S., & Lieberman, L. D. (2020). Three decades of research: The case for comprehensive sex education. *Journal of Adolescent Health*, 68(1), 13–27. 10.1016/j.jadohealth.2020.07.036

Gorman, D. M. (1998). The irrelevance of evidence in the development of school-based drug prevention policy, 1986-1996. *Evaluation Review*, 22(1), 118–146. 10.1177/0193841X9802200106

Hale, D. R., Fitzgerald-Yau, N., & Viner, R. M. (2014). A systematic review of effective interventions for reducing multiple health risk behaviors in adolescence. *American Journal of Public Health*, 104(5), e19–e41.

Hall, W. J., Jones, B. L. H., Witkemper, K. D., Collins, T. L., & Rodgers, G. K. (2019). State policy on school-based sex education: A content analysis focused on sexual behaviors, relationships, and identities. *American Journal of Health Behavior*, 43(3), 506–519. 10.5993/AJHB.43.3.6

Hansen, W. B., & McNeal, R. B. (1997). How D.A.R.E. works: An examination of program effects on mediating variables. *Health Education & Behavior*, 24(2), 165–176. 10.1177/109019819702400205

Harmon, M. A. (1993). Reducing the risk of drug involvement among early adolescents: An evaluation of drug abuse resistance education (DARE. *Evaluation Review*, 17(2), 221–239. 10.1177/0193841X9301700206

Hawkins, R. P., & Vraga, E. (2018). *Evidence-based behavioral models and Fatal Vision Goggles*. Retrieved from fatalvision.com

Heels, S. (2019). The impact of abstinence-only sex education programs in the United States on adolescent sexual outcomes. *Perspectives, 11*(1). https://scholars.unh.edu/perspectives/vol11/iss1/3

Hennessy, D. A., Lanni-Manley, E., & Maiorana, N. (2006). The effects of fatal vision goggles on drinking and driving intentions in college students. *Journal of Drug Education, 36*(1), 59–72. 10.2190/ETB8-3X5W-14K1-EL4R

Herrman, J. W., Waterhouse, J. K., & Chiquoine, J. (2011). Evaluation of an infant simulator intervention for teen pregnancy prevention. *Journal of Obstetric, Gynecologic & Neonatal Nursing, 40*(3), 322–328. 10.1111/j.1552-6909.2011.01248.x

Hoyt, H. H., & Broom, B. L. (2002). School-based teen pregnancy prevention programs: A review of the literature. *The Journal of School Nursing, 18*(1), 11–17. 10.1177/10598405020180010401

Imber, M. (1982). Toward a theory of curriculum reform: An analysis of the first campaign for sex education. *Curriculum Inquiry, 12*(4), 339–362.

Ingraham, C. (2017, June 12). *A brief history of DARE, the anti-drug program Jeff Sessions wants to revive—The Washington Post.* https://www.washingtonpost.com/news/wonk/wp/2017/07/12/a-brief-history-of-d-a-r-e-the-anti-drug-program-jeff-sessions-wants-to-revive/

Irwin, C., Desbrow, B., & McCartney, D. (2019). Effects of alcohol intoxication goggles (fatal vision goggles) with a concurrent cognitive task on simulated driving performance. *Traffic Injury Prevention, 20*(8), 777–782. 10.1080/15389588.2019.1669023

Jewell, J. D., Axelrod, M. I., Prinstein, M. J., & Hupp, S. (2018). *Great myths of adolescence.* John Wiley & Sons.

Jewell, J., & Hupp, S. D. A. (2005). Examining the effects of fatal vision goggles on changing attitudes and behaviors related to drinking and driving. *Journal of Primary Prevention, 26*(6), 553–565. 10.1007/s10935-005-0013-9

Jewell, J., Hupp, S., & Luttrell, G. (2004). The effectiveness of fatal vision goggles: The effectiveness of fatal vision goggles: Disentangling experiential versus onlooker effects. *Journal of Alcohol and Drug Education, 48*(3), 63–84.

jrray. (2016, September 30). *Fatal Vision [Text].* University of Minnesota, Morris. https://morris.umn.edu/morris-public-safety/programs-and-services/fatal-vision

Kirby, D. B. (2008). The impact of abstinence and comprehensive sex and STD/HIV education programs on adolescent sexual behavior. *Sexuality Research & Social Policy, 5*(3), 18. 10.1525/srsp.2008.5.3.18

Kohler, P. K., Manhart, L. E., & Lafferty, W. E. (2008). Abstinence-only and comprehensive sex education and the initiation of sexual activity and teen pregnancy. *Journal of Adolescent Health, 42*(4), 344–351. 10.1016/j.jadohealth.2007.08.026

Kolbe, L. J., Kann, L., & Collins, J. L. (1993). Overview of the youth risk behavior surveillance system. *Public Health Reports, 108*(Suppl 1), 2.

Kralewski, J., & Stevens-Simon, C. (2000). Does mothering a doll change teens' thoughts about pregnancy?. *Pediatrics, 105*(3), e30. 10.1542/peds.105.3.e30

Leeland, J. (2019, June 14). *Bringing up robot baby, a teenage rite of passage*. The New York Times. https://www.nytimes.com/2019/06/14/nyregion/realcare-baby-infant-simulator.html

Leung, H., Shek, D. T. L., Leung, E., & Shek, E. Y. W. (2019). Development of contextually-relevant sexuality education: Lessons from a comprehensive review of adolescent sexuality education across cultures. *International Journal of Environmental Research and Public Health*, 16(4), Article 4. 10.3390/ijerph 16040621

Lindberg, L. D., Firestein, L., & Beavin, C. (2021). Trends in U.S. adolescent sexual behavior and contraceptive use, 2006-2019. *Contraception: X*, 3, 100064. 10.1016/j.conx.2021.100064

Lindberg, L. D., & Maddow-Zimet, I. (2012). Consequences of sex education on teen and young adult sexual behaviors and outcomes. *Journal of Adolescent Health*, 51(4), 332–338. 10.1016/j.jadohealth.2011.12.028

Lynam, D. R., Milich, R., Zimmerman, R., Novak, S. P., Logan, T. K., Martin, C., Leukefeld, C., & Clayton, R. (1999). Project DARE: No effects at 10-year follow-up. *Journal of Consulting and Clinical Psychology*, 67, 590–593. 10.1037/0022-006X.67.4.590

Marlow, K., & Rhodes, S. (1994). Study: DARE teaches kids about drugs but doesn't prevent use. *Herald-Journal*, A3. https://news.google.com/newspapers?nid=1876&dat=19941106&id=EbQeAAAAIBAJ&sjid=Rs8EAAAAIBAJ&pg=6923,1403055

McCartney, D., Desbrow, B., & Irwin, C. (2017). Using alcohol intoxication goggles (Fatal Vision® goggles) to detect alcohol-related impairment in simulated driving. *Traffic Injury Prevention*, 18(1), 19–27. 10.1080/15389588.2016.1190015

Meeker, M., & Kehl, L. (2020, May 4). Substance use: Are specialized goggles effective at preventing impaired driving?. *Sketical Inquirer*, 44(3). https://skepticalinquirer.org/2020/05/dubious-claims-in-psychotherapy-for-youth-part-iii-externalizing-issues-and-daily-routines/

Miech, R., Patrick, M. E., Keyes, K., O'Malley, P. M., & Johnston, L. (2021). Adolescent drug use before and during U.S. national COVID-19 social distancing policies. *Drug and Alcohol Dependence*, 226, 108822. 10.1016/j.drugalcdep.2021.108822

Miller-Day, M., & Hecht, M. L. (2017). Comment to Caputi and McLellan: Truth and D.A.R.E.: Is D.A.R.E.'s new Keepin' it REAL curriculum suitable for American nationwide implementation?. *Drugs: Education, Prevention and Policy*, 24(2), 224–225. 10.1080/09687637.2017.1288685

Morales, A. C., & Day, J. (2017). *The Effects of a Fatal Vision Goggles Intervention on Middle School Aged Children's Attitudes towards Drinking and Driving and Texting while driving* (Doctoral dissertation, Brenau University).

Nasco Education (Director). (2022, February 7). *Fatal Vision Impairment Goggles: The best way to teach students about alcohol and drugs*. https://www.youtube.com/watch?v=jo8csXHTMJ4

Out, J. W., & Lafreniere, K. D. (2001). Baby think it over: Using role-play to prevent teen pregnancy. *Adolescence, 36*(143), 571–582.

Ringwalt, C., Ennett, S. T., & Holt, K. D. (1991). An outcome evaluation of Project DARE (Drug Abuse Resistance Education). *Health Education Research,* 6(3), 327–337. 10.1093/her/6.3.327

Rosenbaum, D. P. (2007, November 29). *Just say no to D.A.R.E.* https:// onlinelibrary.wiley.com/doi/10.1111/j.1745-9133.2007.00474.x

Rosenbaum, D. P., & Hanson, G. S. (1998). Assessing the effects of school-based drug education: A six-year multilevel analysis of project D.A.R.E. *Journal of Research in Crime and Delinquency, 35*(4), 381–412.

Santelli, J., Ott, M. A., Lyon, M., Rogers, J., & Summers, D. (2006). Abstinence-only education policies and programs: A position paper of the Society for Adolescent Medicine. *Journal of Adolescent Health, 38*(1), 83–87. 10.1016/ j.jadohealth.2005.06.002

Santelli, J., Ott, M. A., Lyon, M., Rogers, J., Summers, D., & Schleifer, R. (2006). Abstinence and abstinence-only education: A review of U.S. policies and programs. *Journal of Adolescent Health, 38*(1), 72–81. 10.1016/j.jadohealth. 2005.10.006

Singh, R. D., Jimerson, S. R., Renshaw, T., Saeki, E., Hart, S. R., Earhart, J., & Stewart, K. (2011). A Summary and synthesis of contemporary empirical evidence regarding the effects of the drug abuse resistance education Program (D.A.R.E.). *Contemporary School Psychology, 15*, 93–102.

Somers, C. L., & Fahlman, M. M. (2001). Effectiveness of the "Baby Think It Over" teen pregnancy prevention program. *Journal of School Health, 71*(5), 188–188.

Somerville, L. H., & Casey, B. (2010). Developmental neurobiology of cognitive control and motivational systems. *Current Opinion in Neurobiology, 20*(2), 236–241. 10.1016/j.conb.2010.01.006

Stanger-Hall, K. F., & Hall, D. W. (2011). Abstinence-only education and teen pregnancy rates: Why we need comprehensive sex education in the US. *PloS One, 6*(10), e24658.

Strachan, W., & Gorey, K. M. (1997). Infant simulator lifespace intervention: Pilot investigation of an adolescent pregnancy prevention program. *Child and Adolescent Social Work Journal, 14*(3), 171–180. 10.1023/A:1024565502423

Substance Abuse and Mental Health Services Administration (US) & Office of the Surgeon General (US) (2016). *Facing addiction in America: The surgeon general's report on alcohol, drugs, and health.* US Department of Health and Human Services. http://www.ncbi.nlm.nih.gov/books/NBK424857/

Tingle, L. R. (2002). Evaluation of the North Carolina "Baby think it over" project. *Journal of School Health, 72*(5), 178–183.

Tipton, E., Hallberg, K., Hedges, L. V., & Chan, W. (2017). Implications of small samples for generalization: Adjustments and rules of thumb. *Evaluation Review,* 41(5), 472–505. 10.1177/0193841X16655665

University of North Carolina at Greensboro (2022). An evaluation of the "D.A.R.E.: Keepin' it REAL" elementary school program executive summary. *Prevention Strategies Inspiring Brighter Futures.* https://dare.org/wp-content/

uploads/DARE-kiR-Elementary-Evaluation-Executive-Summary-FINAL-V.
3c.pdf

Vincus, A. A., Ringwalt, C., Harris, M. S., & Shamblen, S. R. (2010). A short-term, quasi-experimental evaluation of D.A.R.E.'s revised elementary school curriculum. *Journal of Drug Education*, *40*(1), 37–49. 10.2190/DE.40.1.c

West, S. L., & O'Neal, K. K. (2004). Project D.A.R.E. outcome effectiveness revisited. *American Journal of Public Health*, *94*(6), 1027–1029. 10.2105/AJPH.94.6.1027

YRBSS Overview | YRBSS | Adolescent and School Health | CDC. (2020, August 18). https://www.cdc.gov/healthyyouth/data/yrbs/overview.htm

Part III

Assessment

6 Cognitive Assessment

Matthew K. Burns and Jonie B. Welland

The titular character from the 1994 movie *Forrest Gump* is undoubtably memorable. His endearing qualities extend far beyond his proposed intelligence quotient (IQ) of 75. Portrayed as agreeable, trusting, forgiving, empathetic, cooperative, and highly likeable (Manggalasri & Luthfiyati, 2018), Gump's personality contrasts sharply with other notable characters. Consider, for instance, Will Hunting from *Goodwill Hunting*, a self-taught genius burdened with assumed accompanying obsessions and mentally unhealthy characteristics (Mendick & Moreau, 2013), or Sheldon Cooper from the *Big Bang Theory* who boasted an IQ of 187 but was characterized by arrogance, narcissism, and lack of social skills (Stratton, 2016).

These fictional characters portray examples of stereotypes based on cognitive aptitude, but these stereotypes are not limited to fictional TV and movie characters. Teacher perceptions of students, influenced by IQ or perceived high or low cognitive ability, can significantly impact which students are referred for gifted and talented services and the types of instruction employed (Childs & Wooten, 2023).

Cognitive assessments are standardized measures designed to provide information about multiple neuropsychological functions that underlie human function and behavior (Kelso & Tadi 2023). Among these assessments, intelligence tests that report an IQ are the most frequently used by school psychologists, which is a practice that has persisted for decades (Benson et al., 2019). The prevalence of IQ tests in schools can be attributed, in part, to three claims about IQ tests: 1) they provide meaningful information about individual students that can be best understood by analyzing subtest scores from cognitive assessments (Kranzler et al., 2020), 2) this analysis can improve the accuracy of specific learning disability (SLD) identification decisions (Benson et al., 2020), and 3) this analysis can also improve efforts to target intervention (Decker et al., 2013).

DOI: 10.4324/9781003266181-9

Examining the Claims

Description of the Claims

As a school psychology graduate student, this chapter's first author was well trained in the administration and interpretation of IQ tests using the third edition of Sattler's (1988) classic *Assessment of Children* textbook. Table C-13 (pages 824–829) contained a list of subtests from a commonly used IQ test and what each one measured. For example, Sattler purported that the Picture Completion subtest measured perceptual organization, ability to differentiate essential from nonessential details, identification of familiar objects, visual recognition, and concentration on visually perceived material (p. 826). Given the author's interest in academic interventions, he committed the entire six-page table to memory. This level of familiarity soon led to an internship supervisor handing over an IQ test protocol with the instruction to "Sattlerize it," which meant to examine the subtest scores and provide a list of strengths and difficulties.

Sattlerizing IQ subtest scores or engaging in profile analysis remains a common but an increasingly sophisticated practice. *Ipsative analysis* refers to the practice of examining intraindividual patterns presented within the subtests that make up the full-scale or global IQ score to better understand student cognitive abilities. The subtest scores are interpreted by (a) calculating an average subtest score for each test taker and identifying those that are significantly lower (weakness) or significantly higher (strength) than the individual's average score, (b) examining the amount of variability in an individual's profile based on the standard deviation of each person's subtest scores, or (c) comparing each subtest to each other to identify relative strengths and difficulties (Zaboski et al., 2018). More contemporary intelligence theories such as Planning, Attention-Arousal, Simultaneous, and Successive (PASS; Naglieri, 1999) and Cattell-Horn-Carroll (CHC; Schneider & McGrew, 2012) can be used as a framework to better understand what each subtest is designed to measure (Flanagan et al., 2000).

The more sophisticated interpretive frameworks for cognitive assessments are believed to provide a more accurate diagnosis of SLD, conceptualized as unexpected underachievement (Fletcher et al., 2005), which could be explained by the presence of a corresponding weakness in one or more specific cognitive abilities that are correlated to the area of underachievement (McDonough & Flanagan, 2016). Thus, if a student has unexplained underachievement in reading but not math, the student would be expected to also have lower score in a CHC domain that is related to reading such as auditory processing (Flanagan et al., 2006). Moreover, SLD "is presumably caused by cognitive processing weaknesses or deficits" (Flanagan & Alfonso, 2017, p. 436).

The more sophisticated interpretive frameworks for cognitive assessments are also believed to explain differential effects of academic interventions (i.e., what works for one student may not work for another). Advocates for cognitive assessment have long claimed that cognitive function data can explain the difference in intervention effects (Cronbach & Snow, 1977). Specific subtests and factor scores from cognitive assessments correlate better with specific areas of academic achievement than others (Zaboski et al., 2018), and in a manner that is consistent with CHC theory (Cormier et al., 2017). Thus, some researchers have suggested that cognitive assessment data might indicate deficit areas that are causing academic underachievement and improving those cognitive deficits through intervention would enhance academic outcomes (Feifer, 2008; Fiorello et al., 2006).

Critical Examination

Cognitive assessments have been a subject of controversy since their inception. Jensen (1969) and Herrnstein and Murray (1994) present cognitive aptitude as a fixed trait that is almost exclusively influenced by heredity, but recent research questions those claims finding that environmental factors are more important in determining cognitive functioning than once believed (Nisbett, 2013). Moreover, cognitive assessments have long been associated with bias against students of color and other underrepresented groups, which have led to negative consequences such as overrepresentation of students from those groups in special education (Garcia, 2015).

It is also a commonly held belief that cognitive ability predicts educational and career outcomes, leading many to believe that professions such as physicians, lawyers, and engineers possess higher cognitive abilities than laborers. However, Mensa International, the largest and oldest non-profit organization for individuals with high cognitive ability, challenges this notion by boasting a diverse membership including police officers, professors, truck drivers, doctors, manual laborers, glass blowers, scientists, and myriad other professions. Thus, the relationship between cognitive ability and career outcomes is not completely clear. Additionally, data from cognitive assessments may predict academic achievement, but they do a poor job of predicting student response to academic interventions ($r = -.11$, Scholin & Burns, 2012; $r = .08$ to $.27$, Stuebing et al., 2009).

Equally controversial are the claims that cognitive assessments can be examined through ipsative analyses, and that the data enhance SLD identification and intervention design. A survey of over 1300 practicing school psychologists found that 69% regularly conduct ipsative analyses of cognitive assessment subtests (Kranzler et al., 2020) and many use this practice to identify potential interventions for individual students (Benson et al., 2019). Moreover, a review of school psychology SLD identification evaluation reports found that data from cognitive assessments (i.e., crystalized ability and working memory) predicted whether or not a team identified a student as SLD better than rates of growth during an intervention, even though growth rates were required elements of the identification process and cognitive assessments were not (Hajovsky et al., 2022). Next, we will describe the research that questions the three aforementioned claims made about cognitive assessments.

Ipsative Analysis

The practice of interpreting subtest scores from cognitive assessments is as old as cognitive assessments themselves and has been questionable since the beginning (Bray et al., 1998). A special issue of *School Psychology Quarterly* (now *School Psychology*) that was published in 2000 was titled "Cognitive Profile Analysis: A Shared Professional Myth" and included four studies that provided research to refute the validity of the practice (Watkins, 2000). Years later, this practice persists despite repeated attempts by researchers to point out the inherent flaws (McGill et al., 2018).

Cognitive assessments are comprised of subtests that directly measure the discrete abilities that are hypothesized to make up intelligence or global functioning. These subtests are often grouped into factors according to the underlying theory, which are represented by factor, index, or composite scores. Most cognitive assessments result in estimates of global ability that are quite reliable, but the subtests used to derive that global ability estimate are often too unreliable to make decisions about individual test takers. For example, some subtests from the fifth edition of the *Wechsler Intelligence Scale for Children* (Wechsler, 2014) resulted in reliability estimates that were quite low (e.g., .67 for Symbol Search), especially for some groups of test takers (e.g., .67 for Matrix Reasoning with students with reading disabilities), and mean test-retest reliabilities were as low as .71 (Picture Concepts; Olivier et al., 2018).

Comparisons of subtests to each other result in multiple comparisons that increase the likelihood of a finding due to error. For example, consider a cognitive assessment that has 10 subtests, all of which are compared to each other, and two are found to be significantly different to $p < .05$. The comparison of all the subtests results in 9 comparisons, then 8, then 7, then 6, etc., which is 45 comparisons. If we randomly assigned scores to the 45 subtests, we would likely find two comparisons that are different to .05. To be sure that the difference is significant, the significance level needed to identify a significant difference between two subtests should be corrected with a Bonferroni adjustment, which is simply the alpha level needed for significance (.05) divided by the number of comparisons (45). In this example, an alpha level less than .001 would be needed to find significance. If there were 14 subtests, then that would be 105 comparisons and the adjusted alpha level would be .0005. Even only four subtests or factor/index/composite scores would require an adjusted alpha level of .005. It is quite possible that conclusions from subtest comparisons are due to error, as currently it is not common practice to conduct a Bonferroni adjustment to determine the significance level.

Even comparisons of composite scores can be questionable, because they do not have sufficient temporal stability (e.g., test-retest reliability .65 to .76; Watkins & Smith, 2013) and large differences in factor, index, or composite scores are likely to reduce over time due to simple regression to the mean (McGill et al., 2018). Thus, the standard errors and resulting confidence intervals for subtest scores and index scores can be quite large, which would make most conclusions drawn from comparisons to be the result of measurement error rather than real differences in student functioning (Canivez, 2013; McGill et al., 2018). Moreover, factor analyses of cognitive assessment data have frequently questioned the proposed structure represented by subtest, factor scores, and composites (Canivez et al., 2017; Styck & Watkins, 2016), which could suggest that practitioners should not have confidence that the purported meaning of the factor, index, or composite score (e.g., Fluid Reasoning may not actually assess the ability to solve problems in new situations; de Jong, in press).

In addition to the psychometric issues previously described, analyzing the subtests or other intraindividual profiles within cognitive assessment can also lead to erroneous decisions if the interpretive framework does not consider the base rate at which the profile exists. A base rate represents the percentage of the population that exhibits the condition being assessed. For example, if 15% of the population had SLD, then any deviation from 15% of the sample being diagnosed with SLD would be error, and high or low base rates can significantly affect the accuracy of the interpretation with low base rates suggesting the possibility of false positives and high base rates making frequent false negatives possible (VanDerHeyden, 2011). Watkins et al. (2022) examined profile analyses for cognitive assessments and found at least one "rare and unusual" ($\geq$ 21-point difference; Kaufman et al., 2016, p. 242) subtest score differences for 24%–28% of the profiles they examined, which is hardly rare or unusual. The high base rate of the profile suggests that it likely represents a point on the continuum of normalcy and interpreting the data would likely lead to erroneous decisions.

Identifying SLD

Federal special education law defines SLD as, "a disorder in one or more of the basic psychological processes involved in understanding or in using language, spoken or written, that may manifest itself in the imperfect ability to listen, think, speak, read, write, spell, or to do mathematical calculations" (Sec. 300.8(c) (10), Individuals with Disabilities Education Act, 2004). Given that the very definition of SLD involves psychological processes, it makes sense to measure them with cognitive assessments when evaluating a student for SLD. However, the federal regulations that operationally define SLD and how to assess for it do not refer to cognitive assessment in any way, except to say that states cannot "require the use of a severe discrepancy between intellectual ability and achievement for determining whether a child has a specific learning disability" (Sec. 300.307). Moreover, the U.S. Department of Education provided guidance to the regulations for implementing special education law and explicitly stated that, "The Department does not believe that an assessment of psychological or cognitive processing should be required in determining whether a child has an SLD. There is no current evidence that such assessments are necessary or sufficient for identifying SLD. Furthermore, in many cases, these assessments have not been used to make appropriate intervention decisions" (IDEA Regulations, 2006, p. 46651). Simply put, there is no mandate to include cognitive assessments in SLD identification.

Hale et al. (2008) concluded that significant intraindividual subtest scatter on cognitive assessments is the hallmark of SLD, and subtest profiles were shown to be correlated to specific types of SLD (Feifer et al., 2014). Notwithstanding the evidence that psychometric difficulties make any application of interpreting cognitive assessment profiles questionable, this specific question has been studied numerous times with alarming results. Extant research regarding the use of cognitive assessment profiles to identify SLD found that identification decisions were not consistent across identification frameworks (Miciak et al., 2015, 2016), and using profile analysis of cognitive assessment data in SLD identification consistently demonstrates poor accuracy (Miciak et al., 2018). More specifically, individual profiles from cognitive assessments did not predict SLD better than chance (McGill, 2018) and resulted in a high false positive rate in which students would be overidentified as having an SLD (Stuebing et al., 2012). Part of the difficulty in validating a model of using cognitive assessment data to identify SLD is that there are a number of models to choose from, and no specific individual profile has been confirmed to identify SLD (Mather & Schneider, 2015). Readers are referred to an excellent article by McGill et al. (2018) that summarizes the history and current and future problems associated with the common practice of interpreting profiles from cognitive assessments.

Targeting Intervention Efforts

Data from cognitive assessments have been suggested as a method for assessing students' academic difficulties and selecting appropriate interventions (Feifer, 2008; Mather & Wendling, 2018). This practice primarily relies on observed correlations between specific subtests or indices and measures of academic achievement (Johnson, 2014). Among the various interesting claims associated with cognitive assessments, the proposed use of these data to guide academic interventions could be viewed as perplexing for optimists, or as problematic, questionable, and harmful for those adopting a more skeptical perspective. Even the researcher who initially advocated for the use of cognitive assessment data in selecting academic interventions renounced this assertion after devoting an entire career to its study (Chronbach & Snow, 1977).

Miciak et al. (2016) examined the profiles from cognitive assessments for 203 fourth-grade students and found that they did not predict response to intensive reading interventions. Multiple meta-analyses also found small effects for selecting academic interventions from cognitive assessments. For example, Burns (2016) found a small effect ($g = 0.17$) for interventions that were selected based on data from cognitive measures, as did Stuebing et al. (2009, 2015). In fact, Burns (2016) reviewed over 200 studies from 7 meta-analyses and found an overall small effect ($d = 0.27$) and concluded that, "Examining cognitive processing data does not improve intervention effectiveness, and doing so could distract attention from more effective interventions" (p. 27).

Some might suggest that there are studies that support using cognitive assessment data to plan interventions, but Schneider and Kaufman (2017) reviewed the research and concluded that, "this position is mostly backed by rhetoric in which assertions are backed by citations of other scholars making assertions backed by citations of still other scholars making assertions" (p. 8). It is not often that researchers can clearly say that empirical data have all but conclusively answered a specific question, but this might be one of those times. Practitioners who use cognitive assessments to select, plan, or monitor academic interventions seem to be prioritizing professional beliefs over scientific findings.

What To Do Instead

Cognitive assessments will probably always have a role in school-based assessments of special education disabilities. For example, a cognitive assessment is likely needed to identify or rule out an intellectual disability, but practitioners should recognize the limits of cognitive assessments and should be careful to not overinterpret the data. Moreover, the score that represents the estimate of global functioning will always be the most reliable and validated score from any cognitive measure and should be either the primary or sole score interpreted.

Ongoing research continues to demonstrate the positive effects of selecting reading and math interventions based on measures of the specific skill needing additional support (Burns, 2021; Burns et al., in press, 2022; Szadokierski et al., 2017), which is called a skill-by-treatment interaction (Burns et al., 2010). The best assessment approach to identify a reading intervention that is appropriate for an individual student is to assess reading with that student, and then select interventions with well-documented positive effects.

Summary and Conclusion

It is difficult to understand how questionable claims about cognitive assessment persist in the face of voluminous research. One reason could be because it is advocated for and described in various textbooks about assessment (Flanagan & Alfonso, 2017; Flanagan & Harrison, 2012; Groth-Marnat & Wright, 2016; Kaufman et al., 2016; Sattler, 2008) that are frequently used as authoritative sources of information by school and clinical psychology training programs. Moreover, school psychologists spend most of their time engaged in conducting evaluations to identify special education disabilities, and much of that time is spent conducting cognitive assessments. The well-intentioned practitioner likely believes that interpreting cognitive assessments in a manner that both truly identifies SLD and can provide information for instructional planning adds value to that activity and puts them in a position to own information that is specialized to them.

More importantly, society values cognitive assessments and the information they provide. Psychology was forever changed when Alfred Binet invented the first IQ test in 1905. Although psychology has existed as a field much longer, before 1905 it was more associated with philosophy than science. The advent of intelligence testing helped to move psychology graduate programs at most universities out of philosophy departments and gave the field more tangible and understandable ideas. When parents are given a psychological report about their children they often read the information from cognitive assessments with great interest. Society values the information thought to be provided by cognitive assessments; however, the research does not support the clinical traditions described here.

References

Benson, N. F., Floyd, R. G., Kranzler, J. H., Eckert, T. L., Fefer, S. A., & Morgan, G. B. (2019). Test use and assessment practices of school psychologists in the United States: Findings from the 2017 National Survey. *Journal of School Psychology*, 72, 29–48. 10.1016/j.jsp.2018.12.004

Benson, N. F., Maki, K. E., Floyd, R. G., Eckert, T. L., Kranzler, J. H., & Fefer, S. A. (2020). A national survey of school psychologists' practices in identifying specific learning disabilities. *School Psychology, 35*(2), 146–157. 10.1037/spq0000344

Bray, M. A., Kehle, T. J., & Hintze, J. M. (1998). Profile analysis with the Wechsler Scales: Why does it persist?. *School Psychology International, 19*(3), 209–220.

Burns, M. K. (2016). Effect of cognitive processing assessments and interventions on academic outcomes: Can 200 studies be wrong?. *Communique, 44*(5), 1, 26–29.

Burns, M. K. (2021). Intensifying reading interventions through a skill-by-treatment interaction: What to do when nothing else worked. *NASP Communiqué, 50*(4), 1, 30–32.

Burns, M. K., Codding, R. S., Boice, C. H., & Lukito, G. (2010). Meta-analysis of acquisition and fluency math interventions with instructional and frustration level skills: Evidence for a skill-by-treatment interaction. *School Psychology Review, 39*(1), 69–83.

Burns, M. K., Duesenberg-Marshall, M. D., Sussman-Dawson, K., Romero, M. E., Wilson, D., & Felten, M. (in press). Effects of targeting reading interventions: Testing a skill-by-treatment interaction in an applied setting. *Preventing School Failure.*

Burns, M. K., Young, H., McCollom, E. M., Stevens, M. A., & Izumi, J. (2022). Predicting intervention effects with preintervention measures of decoding: Evidence for a skill-by-treatment interaction with kindergarten and first-grade students. *Learning Disability Quarterly, 45*(4) 320–330. 10.1177/073194 87221113026

Canivez, G. L. (2013). Psychometric versusactuarial interpretation of intelligence and related aptitude batteries. *The Oxford handbook of child psychological assessment,* 84–112.

Canivez, G. L., Watkins, M. W. , & Dombrowski, S. C. (2017). Structural validity of the Wechsler Intelligence Scale for Children-Fifth Edition: Confirmatory factor analyses with the 16 primary and secondary subtests. *Psychological Assessment, 29*(4), 458–472.

Childs, T. M., & Wooten, N. R. (2023). Teacher bias matters: An integrative review of correlates, mechanisms, and consequences. *Race Ethnicity and Education, 26*(3), 368–397. 10.1080/13613324.2022.2122425

Cronbach, L. & Snow, R. (1977). *Aptitudes and instructional methods: A handbook for research on interactions.* New York: Irvington.

Cormier, D. C., McGrew, K. S., Bulut, O., & Funamoto, A. (2017). Revisiting the relations between the WJ-IV measures of Cattell-Horn-Carroll (CHC) cognitive abilities and reading achievement during the school-age years. *Journal of Psychoeducational Assessment, 35*(8), 731–754.

de Jong, P. F. (in press). The validity of WISC-V profiles of strengths and weaknesses. *Journal of Psychoeducational Assessment.* 10.1177/07342829221150868

Decker, S. L., Hale, J. B., & Flanagan, D. P. (2013). Professional practice issues in the assessment of cognitive functioning for educational applications. *Psychology in the Schools, 50*(3), 300–313. 10.1002/pits.21675, 10.1080/21622965.2014.993396

Feifer, S. G. (2008). Integrating Response to Intervention (RTI) with neuropsychology: A scientific approach to reading. *Psychology in the Schools*, 45(9), 812–825.

Feifer, S. G., Nader, R. G., Flanagan, D., Fitzer, K. R., & Hicks, K. (2014). Identifying specific reading disability subtypes for effective educational remediation. *Learning Disabilities: A Multidisciplinary Journal*, 20(1), 18–31.

Fiorello, C. A., Hale, J. B., & Snyder, L. E. (2006). Cognitive hypothesis testing and response to intervention for children with reading problems. *Psychology in the Schools*, 43(8), 835–853.

Flanagan, D. P. (2000). Wechsler-based CHC cross-battery assessment and reading achievement: Strengthening the validity of interpretations drawn from Wechsler test scores. *School Psychology Quarterly*, 15(3), 295–329. 10.1037/h0088789

Flanagan, D. P., & Alfonso, V. C. (2017). *Essentials of WISC-V assessment*. John Wiley & Sons.

Flanagan, D. P., & Harrison, P. L. (Eds.). (2012). *Contemporary intellectual assessment: Theories, tests, and issues* (3rd ed.). Guilford.

Flanagan, D. P., Ortiz, S. O., Alfonso, V. C., & Mascolo, J. T. (2006). *The achievement test desk reference: A guide to learning disability identification*. John Wiley & Sons Incorporated.

Fletcher, J. M., Denton, C., & Francis, D. J. (2005). Validity of alternative approaches for the identification of learning disabilities: Operationalizing unexpected underachievement. *Journal of Learning Disabilities*, 38(6), 545–552.

Garcia, E. (2015). Lorenzo P. v. Riles? Should the" Larry P." Prohibitions be extended to english language learners?: Considering public policy & IQ testing in schools. *Multicultural Education*, 22(2), 2–7.

Groth-Marnat, G., & Wright, A. J. (2016). *Handbook of psychological assessment* (6th ed.). John Wiley & Sons.

Hajovsky, D. B., Maki, K. E., Chesnut, S. R., Barrett, C. A., & Burns, M. K. (2022). Specific learning disability identification in an RtI method: Do measures of cognitive ability matter?. *Learning Disabilities Research & Practice*, 37(4), 280–293. 10.1111/ldrp.12292

Hale, J. B., Flanagan, D. P., & Naglieri, J. A. (2008). Alternative research-basedm ethodsfor IDEA (2004) identification of children with specific learning disabilities. *Communique*, 36(8), 14–17.

Herrnstein, R. J. & Murray, C. (1994). *The bell curve: Intelligence and class structure in American life*. The Free Press.

Individuals with Disabilities Education Act (2004). 20 U.S.C. § 1400.

Individuals with Disabilities Education Act (IDEA) regulations 34 C.F.R. §§ 300.3 et seq (2006). IDEA regulations commentary, 71 Fed. Reg. 46651, (2006, August 14). Available at http://idea.ed.gov/download/finalregulations.pdf

Jensen, A. R. (1969). How much can we boost IQ and scholastic achievement?. *Harvard Educational Review*, 39, 1–123.

Johnson, E. S. (2014). Understanding why a child is struggling to learn: The role of cognitive processing evaluation in learning disability identification. *Topics in Language Disorders*, 34(1), 59–73. DOI: 10.1097/TLD.0000000000000007

Kaufman, A. S., Raiford, S. E., & Coalson, D. L. (2016). *Intelligent testing with the WISC-V*. Wiley.

Kelso, I. G. & Tadi, P. (2023). *Cognitive assessment*. National Center for Biotechnical Information. Available online at https://www.ncbi.nlm.nih.gov/books/NBK55 6049/#:~:text=Definition%2FIntroduction,during%20the%20Mental%20Status %20Exam.

Kranzler, J. H., Maki, K. E., Benson, N. F., Eckert, T. L., Floyd, R. G., & Fefer, S. A. (2020). How do school psychologists interpret intelligence tests for the identification of specific learning disabilities?. *Contemporary School Psychology*, *24*, 445–456. 10.1007/s40688-020-00274-0

Manggalasari, D. S., & Luthfiyati, D. (2018). An analysis of the character of Forrest Gump movie by Robert Zemeckis viewed from Big Five personality traits theory. *E-Link Journal*, *5*(2), 89–92. DOI: 10.30736/ej.v5i2.65

Mather, N., & Schneider, D. (2015). The use of intelligence tests in the diagnosis of specific reading disability. In S. Goldstein, D. Princiotta, & J. A. Naglieri (Eds.). *Handbook of intelligence: Evolutionary theory, historical perspective, and current concepts* (pp. 415–433). Springer.

Mather, N. , & Wendling, B. J. (2018). Linking cognitive abilities to academic interventions for students with specific learning disabilitiesIn D. P. Flanagan & E. M. McDonough (Eds.), *Contemporary intellectual assessment: Theories, tests, and issues*(pp. 777–809). The Guilford Press.

McDonough, E. M., & Flanagan, D. P. (2016). Use of the Woodcock–Johnson IV in the identification of specific learning disabilities in school-age children. In *WJ IV Clinical Use and Interpretation* (pp. 211–252). Academic Press.

McGill, R. J. (2018) Confronting the base rate problem: More ups and downs for cognitive scatter analysis. *Contemporary School Psychology*, *22*, 384–393. 10. 1007/s40688-017-0168-4

McGill, R. J., Dombrowski, S. C., & Canivez, G. L. (2018). Cognitive profile analysis in school psychology: History, issues, and continued concerns. *Journal of School Psychology*, *71*, 108–121. 10.1016/j.jsp.2018.10.007

Mendick, H., & Moreau, M. P. (2013). From good will hunting to deal or no deal: Using popular culture in the mathematics classroom. In D. Leslie & H. Mendick (Eds.) *Debates in mathematics education* (pp. 37–46). Routledge.

Miciak, J., Taylor, W. P., Denton, C. A., & Fletcher, J. M. (2015). The effect of achievement test selection on identification of learning disabilities within a patterns of strengths and weaknesses framework. *School Psychology Quarterly*, *30*, 321–334. 10.1037/spq0000091.

Miciak, J., Taylor, W. P., Stuebing, K. K., & Fletcher, J. M. (2018). Simulation of LD identification accuracy using a pattern of processing strengths and weaknesses method with multiple measures. *Journal of Psychoeducational Assessment*, *36*, 21–33. 10.1177/0734282916683287.

Miciak, J., Williams, J. L., Taylor, W. P., Cirino, P. T., Fletcher, J. M., & Vaughn, S. (2016). Do patterns of strengths and weaknesses predict differential treatment response?. *Journal of Educational Psychology*, *108*, 898–909. 10.1037/ edu0000096.

Naglieri, J. A. (1999). *Essentials of CAS assessment*. Wiley.

Nisbett, R. E. (2013). Schooling makes you smarter: What teachers need to know about IQ. *American Educator*, *37*(1), 10.

Olivier, T. W., Mahone, M., & Jacobson, L. A. (2018). Weschler intelligence scale for children. In J. Kreutzer, J. DeLuca, B. Caplan (Eds.), *Encyclopedia of clinical neuropsychology* (pp. 1–8). Springer. 10.1007/978-3-319-56782-2_1605-2

Sattler, J. M. (1988). *Assessment of children.*

Sattler, J. M. (2008). *Assessment of children: Cognitive foundations.*

Schneider, W. J., & Kaufman, A. S. (2017). Let's not do away with comprehensive cognitive assessments just yet. *Archives of Clinical Neuropsychology, 32,* 8–20. DOI: 10.1093/arclin/acw104.

Schneider, W. J., & McGrew, K. S. (2012). The Cattell-Horn-Carroll model of intelligence. In D. P. Flanagan, & P. L. Harrison (Eds.). *Contemporary intellectual assessment: Theories, tests, and issues* (pp. 99–144). (3rd ed.). Guilford.

Scholin, S. E., & Burns, M. K. (2012). Relationship between pre-intervention data and post-intervention reading fluency and growth: A meta-analysis of assessment data for individual students. *Psychology in the Schools, 49*(4), 385–398.

Stuebing, K. K., Barth, A. E., Molfese, P. J., Weiss, B., & Fletcher, J. M. (2009). IQ is not strongly related to response to reading instruction: A meta-analytic interpretation. *Exceptional Children, 76*(1), 31–51.

Stuebing, K. K., Barth, A. E., Trahan, L. H., Reddy, R. R., Miciak, J., & Fletcher, J. M. (2015). Are child cognitive characteristics strong predictors of responses to intervention? A meta-analysis. *Review of Educational Research, 85*(3), 395–429. DOI: 10.3102/0034654314555996

Stuebing, K. K., Fletcher, J. M., Branum-Martin, L., Francis, D. J., & VanDerHeyden, A. (2012). Evaluation of the technical adequacy of three methods for identifying specific learning disabilities based on cognitive discrepancies. *School Psychology Review, 41*(1), 3–22. 10.1080/02796015. 2012.12087373

Styck, K. M., & Watkins, M. W. (2016). Structural validity of the WISC-IV for students with learning disabilities. *Journal of Learning Disabilities, 49*(2), 216–224.

Stratton, J. (2016): Die Sheldon die: The Big Bang Theory, everyday neoliberalism and Sheldon as neoliberal man, *Journal for Cultural Research,* DOI: 10.1080/14797585.2015.1123515

Szadokierski, I., Burns, M. K., & McComas, J. J. (2017). Predicting intervention effectiveness from reading accuracy and rate measures through the instructional hierarchy: Evidence for a skill-by-treatment interaction. *School Psychology Review, 46*(2), 190–200.

VanDerHeyden, A. M. (2011). Technical adequacy of response to intervention decisions. *Exceptional Children, 77*(4), 335–350. doi: 10.1177/0014402911 07700305

Watkins, M. W. (2000). Cognitive profile analysis: A shared professional myth. *School Psychology Quarterly, 15*(4), 465–479. 10.1037/h0088802

Watkins, M. W., & Smith, L. G. (2013). Long-term stability of the Wechsler Intelligence Scale for Children--Fourth Edition. *Psychological Assessment, 25*(2), 477–483.

Watkins, M. W., Canivez, G. L., Dombrowski, S. C., McGill, R. J., Pritchard, A. E., Holingue, C. B., & Jacobson, L. A. (2022). Long-term stability of Wechsler

Intelligence Scale for Children–fifth edition scores in a clinical sample. *Applied Neuropsychology: Child, 11*(3), 422–428. 10.1080/21622965.2021.1875827

Wechsler, D. (2014). *Wechsler intelligence scale for children* (5th ed.). NCS Pearson.

Zaboski II, B. A., Kranzler, J. H., & Gage, N. A. (2018). Meta-analysis of the relationship between academic achievement and broad abilities of the Cattell-Horn-Carroll theory. *Journal of School Psychology, 71*, 42–56.

7 Academic Assessment

Jeremy Miciak, Ryan L. Famer, and Amanda M. VanDerHeyden

Educational achievement directly impacts student's future opportunities and success. It is widely recognized that a student's academic achievement in primary and secondary grades can have a major impact on their ability to secure admission to college, obtain scholarships, and access well-paying careers. School psychologists have long been integral to assessing students' reading, writing, and math skills when they struggle in school. Assessment is a critical component of the instructional process and can serve multiple purposes. Educators can use assessment data on an individual student's current knowledge and skills for *formative* purposes to make midstream adjustments to instruction (e.g., intensify or de-intensify intervention support) and instructional decision-making (e.g., resource allocation, program evaluation). Educators can also use assessment data for *summative* purposes to determine whether the student has learned key content or skills. Additionally, in the context of special services and interventions, assessment data can be used for individual *identification*, understood broadly as a process to identify risk or more formally to identify a student with a disability in need of protections afforded under multiple federal laws. Despite these differences in how assessment data may be used for educational decision-making, there are specific considerations required to ensure we are implementing a fair and equitable assessment process with evidence for the validity and reliability of our decision-making framework. Assessment cannot meet the standards of fair, equitable, reliable, and valid in educational contexts if it is not situated in (and therefore useful for) informing instruction. Assessment should never occur in a vacuum, nor should we consider or discuss assessment outside the context of how the data obtained will inform instruction. In this chapter, we will examine several claims related to assessment and the assessment process in K-12 settings.

Examining the Claims

Several claims related to academic assessment are based on misconceptions rooted in long-standing pseudoscientific understandings of instruction and

DOI: 10.4324/9781003266181-10

learning (e.g., learning styles, aptitude-by-treatment interactions [ATIs]), whereas others are rooted in more benign misconceptions of the purpose and limitations of the assessment process. We will focus on discussing the common misconceptions that are at the root of these unsupported claims. As we present, rebuke, and correct these misconceptions, readers will detect a common theme: assessment is an imperfect process that always occurs in an instructional context. When we, as educators, fully embrace this reality, a number of core recommendations for improving the assessment process become immediately apparent:

1 **Assessment should be a holistic process.** Validity is not an inherent attribute of a test or process. Instead, validity must be considered holistically as an evaluation of the procedures, decision-making framework, and consequences of those decisions (Kane, 2013; Messick, 1986). With this in mind, we must broaden our discussion of assessment beyond "test validity" and fully consider the instructional consequences of the assessment process, score interpretation, and the decisions and actions that do or do not follow.

2 **Assessment should be recursive.** No test is perfect; all tests suffer from imperfect reliability and none perfectly measure the attribute of interest (e.g., reading, math reasoning). With this in mind, assessment processes must be built to be robust to these errors in measurement. Generally, this means that processes should include multiple assessments administered contextually to address suspected limitations (e.g., following specific intervals of instructional changes) and consider confidence intervals in score interpretations.

3 **Assessment should reflect instructional priorities.** There are few natural constraints on the skills and knowledge we may wish to assess. However, there are considerable, important constraints on what we have the time and capacity to assess in routine practice, particularly when considering processes for universal screening. Assessment decisions always represent a declaration of priorities. Thus, assessment processes should directly measure key academic knowledge and skills, rather than tangential, often weakly related correlates or presumed causes of academic difficulties. Allocating assessment time to lower-priority targets not only wastes resources, but it also invites decision errors because all assessments carry risk of error.

In the sections that follow, we discuss nine common misconceptions that we have encountered in educational practice and research. Many of these misconceptions are rooted in misunderstandings of the broad constructs of test reliability and validity, which inform the confidence afforded the educational decisions we make based on test data. Other misconceptions are rooted in recommendations about what academic skills should be assessed and in what way. Additionally, in recognition of the intrinsic link between assessment and the instructional context in which it occurs, we discuss important misconceptions about instructional opportunity and instructional recommendations for struggling readers based on assessment data. As we delve into the specific misconceptions that can arise in our field, it is important to keep in mind that our list is not exhaustive, and that scientific knowledge continues to evolve. By confronting these misconceptions head-on, we can improve the likelihood that our practices are evidence-based, effective, and ethical. This is particularly crucial in educational services, where the well-being and success of students are at stake. Through a commitment to identifying and dismissing ineffective practices and beliefs about how students learn, we can work toward providing the highest quality education possible.

Misconception #1: A Test Can Be Reliable and Valid across All Contexts

It is common when considering test selection to discuss the reliability and validity of a test, as if these constructs are inherent properties of the test, independent of the instructional context in which we administer the test. In fact, the consideration of reliability and validity for educational tests must always occur in a specific instructional context, framed around the instructional decision that test data inform. This instructional context includes considerations of the child we wish to assess, the instruction they have and will receive, as well as the programmatic changes we might wish to make. For this reason, a test with strong claims to validity in specific contexts might lack such support in other contexts. For example, many early literacy screeners may have strong support for their ability to identify English reading risk among children who speak English as their primary language (January & Klingbeil, 2020; Kilgus et al., 2014). However, we may need to exercise caution in interpreting those data in the same way for a child who is learning English as a second language and who has received little English instruction (Newell et al., 2020). Another very common example is concluding that a child is displaying academic risk because the child has scored below a national normative cut-off criterion without regard to how that student's peers in the same instructional context perform. Evidence to support the validity of a score is necessarily attached to and situated in the instructional context in which the score was collected. The context and proposed use of test data must always be considered when discussing claims of reliability and validity.

Misconception #2: Academic Screening Tests Are Stable across Contexts

One of the most common misconceptions when evaluating academic screening tests is to treat classification accuracy as a unidimensional construct. Within this view, the goal is to choose a screening measure that maximizes "accuracy," often using a single metric such as overall accuracy or Area Under the Curve. However, accuracy is not unidimensional and error types must be carefully considered in their instructional context, particularly because there are inherent tradeoffs between error types. Typically, test accuracies are characterized by sensitivity and specificity. Sensitivity is the proportion of criterion-positive cases (i.e., true cases of the disorder) that are detected by the assessment. Specificity is the proportion of the criterion-negative cases (i.e., individuals who do not have the disorder) that are detected by the assessment. Because of the nature of the variables (binary) and the calculation of the metrics, gaining specificity generally means making the test easier to pass, which necessarily weakens sensitivity. Similarly, gaining sensitivity generally means making the test easier to fail, which necessarily weakens specificity.

In addition to considering error types and instructional context, one must consider the base rate (i.e., the proportion of the population affected) of the disorder within the assessment context. The base rate fallacy describes a tendency to ignore the prevalence of a disorder in considering the accuracy of a test, for example a screening test to determine which students are at-risk. In actuality, assessment accuracy necessarily and functionally interacts with the prevalence of risk (i.e., the base rate or pre-test probability) to result in differing (often widely differing) ranges of decision accuracy following the use of any assessment. The accuracy that is typically reported as sensitivity and specificity is that which is calculated when the probability of being at-risk is identical to the probability of not being at-risk (i.e., 50% base rate), which is often not the case in academic screening.

Misconception #3: Imperfect Reliability for Individual Decisions Precludes Tiered Support Systems

No test is perfect. Test scores vary based on the characteristics of the individual and the test. For this reason, any dichotomous decision that is based on the application of a strict cut point will demonstrate unreliability at the individual level (Francis et al., 2005; Macmann & Barnett, 1985). This observation is often presented as an argument against the adoption of multi-tiered systems of support (MTSS) (Hale et al., 2010), with opponents arguing there are no agreed-upon methods for identifying inadequate response and that decisions will vary based on measurement occasion and test selection. However, these reliability challenges at the individual level are universal and will be applicable whenever we are forced to make a categorical decision based on imperfect, continuous data. In other words, this limitation of imperfect reliability is not unique nor specific to MTSS, but rather exists in all assessments. Furthermore, the benefit of the opportunity to quantify the exclusionary criterion (i.e., ruling out lack of adequate instruction) by directly optimizing the instruction a child receives and evaluating child response directly as part of the assessment process provides benefits that outweigh this limitation that is inherent to all assessment.

Misconception #4: More Data Naturally Leads to Improved Decisions and Outcomes

Misunderstanding that assessment accuracy is necessarily a function of the accuracy of the measure and the context in which you are making a decision often leads teams to collect data points that do not optimally inform screening decisions. For example, it is common for decision-making teams to collect duplicative screening data. This collection of multiple data points to reach a screening decision used to be popularly recommended as a necessary feature of ensuring the reliability of scores. In fact, many readers will recall the early recommendations in curriculum-based measurement to collect three reading CBM scores and record the median value for decision-making. In reality, well-designed academic screening measures generally yield highly correlated scores (Ardoin et al., 2004). In fact, demonstrating concurrent correlation evidence is one way new assessments are validated for practical use. Thus, administering multiple measures with highly correlated scores concurrently is not likely to improve the reliability of the decision in a meaningful way. Instead, additional data often force teams to reconcile potentially disparate scores, creating confusion and delaying instructional action-taking. Overzealous academic screening has been ubiquitous in many schools with most children receiving multiple screening measures at several time points. In recent years, many schools have adopted overlapping screening procedures in response to dyslexia screening laws, in which schools successively screen for reading risk in MTSS and reading risk for dyslexia programs. Yet, there is a point of diminishing returns in academic screening that is rapidly reached and additional screening beyond that point is generally not only helpful but costs instructional time and can worsen learning (VanDerHeyden et al., 2018). Broadly speaking, collecting additional sources of data that are not uniquely information-rich (i.e., are non-diagnostic) is likely to waste precious resources, reduce opportunities for more effective assessment and/or instruction, and may hinder effective decision-making (Dombrowski et al. 2021).

Assessment data alone cannot improve student outcomes; it only affects outcomes through informing instruction. Fundamentally, assessment characterizes what is presently observable which allows us to forecast what performance may look like in the future without intervention, but it tells us nothing of what performance might look like with well-designed and delivered instruction (Miciak et al., 2014, 2016; Stuebing et al., 2009). Given that instructional environments are not stable, it is not possible for assessment alone to improve achievement or close opportunity gaps. Such a statement seems logical, but one of the most resource-consuming activities in schools in the spring is changing screening systems. Most systems would do better instead to process, interpret, and act on their data to intensify instruction. Intensifying instruction is the only way to improve achievement and close opportunity gaps. Tactics like class-wide intervention have shown remarkable promise to improve achievement on proximal and distal measures (VanDerHeyden et al., 2022), to close opportunity gaps (VanDerHeyden & Codding, 2015), and to improve the accuracy of screening decisions to determine who really needs small-group or individual intervention (VanDerHeyden et al., 2021).

Misconception #5: Instruction Should Be Tailored to the Student's Cognitive Profile

A common position among some school psychologists is that a student's cognitive profile – that is, the student's pattern of cognitive strengths and weaknesses – can inform decision makers about the nature of a student's learning difficulties and can aid in intervention selection. This position is based on the ATI paradigm which contends that matching instructional strategy or treatment to the specific aptitude(s) of the student is critical for success. Despite the face validity of this proposal, research efforts to identify specific ATIs have been generally unsuccessful (Burns et al., 2016). One significant issue especially pertaining to the use of cognitive profiles is that students with learning disabilities do not present with consistent cognitive profiles (Watkins & Canivez, 2022). However, it is unclear if our assessment methodologies are simply insufficient to reliably identify cognitive profiles at this time or if there really are no consistent profiles among students with learning disabilities. Regardless of the existence of cognitive profiles for students with learning disabilities, researchers thus far have been unable to develop treatment selection procedures from student neuropsychological data (Burns et al., 2016).

Misconception #6: Strong Core Instruction Is Sufficient to Improve Achievement for All Learners

It seems logical that when a program of instruction is returning weak results that changing the program of instruction will produce an immediate and useful improvement. This logic causes instructional leaders to allocate a great deal of available resources to considering and adopting new programs of instruction. MTSS leaders have often warned implementers that "they cannot intervene their way out of a core instructional problem." This common advice makes sense from an efficiency perspective. In other words, when many students are performing in a risk range, then universal instructional improvements are necessary. Yet, adopting a new curriculum is generally an expensive and low-value tactic because core curricula have relatively weak effect sizes on achievement (e.g., in math, Slavin & Lake, 2008). Evaluation of math curricula, in particular, yields dismal outcomes concerning the extent to which the curricula include principles of effective instructional design (Doabler et al., 2012). Poor outcomes in schools are generally produced over many years of less-than-optimal instruction which includes the local expectations for skill mastery, the consistency and quality of teacher-delivered instruction, the dosage of opportunities to respond, corrective feedback, and supported generalization instruction. Screening data can be used to drive MTSS but they can also be used for ongoing program evaluation so that teams can continually test and refine program improvements with midstream adjustments to attain reduced risk (improved proficiency) and make data-informed resource allocation decisions over time (Kovaleski et al., 2022).

Misconception #7: Instructional Opportunity Is Stable across Classrooms

Instructional opportunity varies across classrooms, with some teachers engineering more effective instruction more consistently than others. To illustrate, consider this quote from Hanushek (2011) discussing differences in learning for students assigned to different teachers:

> … average gains in learning across classrooms, even classrooms within the same school, are very different. Some teachers year after year produce bigger gains in student learning than other teachers. The magnitude of the differences is truly large, with some teachers producing 1.5 years of gain in achievement in an academic year while others with equivalent students produce only ½ year of gain. In other words, two students starting at the same level of achievement can know vastly different amounts at the end of a single academic year due solely to the teacher to which they are assigned. If a bad year is compounded by other bad years, it may not be possible for the student to recover.
>
> (Hanushek, 2011, p. 467).

The instability of instructional quality and effects across classrooms can be detected with academic screening data and year-end test scores, and this instability is deadly to the accuracy of risk decisions that may be based on static screening or year-end test data about students. The likelihood of a false-positive decision error about a child referral is elevated in classrooms in which instruction is weaker (or stated another way, the base rate of risk is higher; VanDerHeyden & Witt, 2005). The only way to remove the error associated with variable instructional quality is to provide an interval of stable instructional quality and evaluate assessment results given adequate instruction.

Misconception #8: Progress Monitoring Data Is Sufficient on Its Own

Data on individual students' rate of improvement is not a panacea for improved educational decision-making, particularly at the individual level. Most reliably, repeated measurement during the school year may provide evidence that instructional effects differ across classrooms, which can guide targeted professional development and instructional modifications. However, rate of improvement in isolation is not sufficient to attribute differences in intervention response to inter-individual differences and make consequential identification decisions (Miciak & Fletcher, 2019; VanDerHeyden & Burns, 2018). There are multiple contextual factors that contribute to variability in observed rates of improvement within a response to intervention framework (Reschly & Coolong-Chaffin, 2016). Most importantly, the quality and consistency of the intervention is the primary driver of the observed rate of improvement. Rate of improvement obtained through progress monitoring can be highly useful given in-tandem evidence that a generally effective intervention was selected and deployed in a high-quality way, but when systems attempt to repeat assessments, calculate rate of improvement, and reach conclusions about growth either via benchmark or normative rates of improvement, conclusions will be highly error-prone because such assessment captures nothing about instructional opportunity.

Misconception #9: Intensifying Instruction Is Only a Matter of Resource Expenditure

Instructional intensification is a relatively new concept in education, gaining popularity as a concept in MTSS frameworks. When MTSS was a new framework, intensification was generally conceptualized as increased time (minutes per session, days per week, and total weeks), more expensive teacher arrangements (e.g., 1:1 as opposed to 1:5 teacher-to-student ratios), and frequency of progress monitoring (Batsche et al., 2006). Over the last two decades, a more sophisticated operationalization of intensification has emerged that emphasizes different characteristics. Specifically, interventions that are developed based on measured student skill proficiencies, that are delivered at a sufficiently frequent dose, that are monitored at least weekly, and that focus on delivering specific instructional tactics that are aligned with student learning needs according to the instructional hierarchy (Haring & Eaton, 1978) are better methods of intensifying instruction than dimensions like time or teacher: student ratios. It turns out that whether an intervention is delivered 1:2 or 1:5 does not change the intensity of the intervention (Clarke et al., 2017; Doabler et al., 2019). Dosage research has demonstrated that more frequently delivered shorter-duration sessions produce stronger gains on learning (Duhon et al., 2022). Other dimensions of intensification include scope of the training set (more narrow scope provides more rapid improvement; Hernandez-Nuhfer et al., 2020) and skill type (more narrowly defined targets produce more rapid growth; Solomon et al., 2020). More frequent progress monitoring is associated with intensification because it can enable dynamic adjustment of the intervention, promote continued alignment of the intervention with student need, and make apparent and thus enable the correction of intervention implementation integrity problems. Though research has provided a more sophisticated understanding of intensification, it also has clarified how difficult it is for teachers to intensify instruction in classrooms (Garet et al., 2008, 2011, 2016). In a series of well-funded studies, Garet and colleagues found that 68–110 hours of summer training, meetings during the school year, and in-class coaching support improved teacher content knowledge in reading and math, but did not improve teacher capacity to make formative adjustments to improve learning. Achievement was unimproved as a result.

Summary and Conclusion

Academic assessment plays a crucial role in the instructional process and is inherently embedded in the instructional environment. For this reason, it is necessary to consider assessment practices *in the context of instruction.* However, many misconceptions have led to a variety of questionably effective practices in school psychology and education that work against many of the goals of educators and school psychologists.

This chapter highlights such misconceptions in the field of academic assessment and instruction, some of which are rooted in pseudoscientific beliefs or simply presented as facts in contradiction to research evidence. Because these beliefs are often taught in undergraduate and graduate programs for educators, educational administrators, school psychologists, and so on, they can become deeply entrenched in school culture, policy, and practice. While it is necessary for school psychologists to be aware of effective and efficient academic assessment and instruction practices, it is also crucial that they be aware of which practices are not validated, ineffective, unnecessary, or harmful (Dombrowski et al., 2021; Travers, 2017). Challenging these misconceptions is critical and requires developing a careful understanding of the variables that maintain their use (Farmer et al., 2021) such that they can be successfully avoided or de-implemented (Shaw, 2021). Reducing the use of questionably effective practices is critical to making the way for evidence-based assessment practices and instruction, and a necessary step to helping students succeed academically.

Author Note. This research was supported by grant P50 HD052117, Texas Center for Learning Disabilities, from the Eunice Kennedy Shriver National Institute of Child Health and Human Development. The content is solely the responsibility of the authors and does not necessarily represent the official views of the Eunice Kennedy Shriver National Institute of Child Health and Human Development or the National Institutes of Health.

References

Ardoin, S. P., Witt, J. C., Suldo, S. M., Connell, J. E., Koenig, J. L., Resetar, J. L., Slider, N. J., & Williams, K. L. (2004). Examining the incremental benefits of administering a maze and three versus one curriculum-based measurement reading probes when conducting universal screening. *School Psychology Review, 33*(2), 218–233. 10.1080/02796015.2004.12086244

Batsche, G. M., Kavale, K. A., & Kovaleski, J. F. (2006). Competing views: A dialogue on response to intervention. *Assessment for Effective Intervention: Official Journal of the Council for Educational Diagnostic Services, 32*(1), 6–19. 10.1177/15345084060320010301

Burns, M. K., Petersen-Brown, S., Haegele, K., Rodriguez, M., Schmitt, B., Cooper, M., ... & VanDerHeyden, A. M. (2016). Meta-analysis of academic interventions derived from neuropsychological data. *School Psychology Quarterly, 31*(1), 28–42.

Clarke, B., Doabler, C. T., Kosty, D., Kurtz Nelson, E., Smolkowski, K., Fien, H., & Turtura, J. (2017). Testing the efficacy of a kindergarten mathematics intervention by small group size. *AERA Open, 3*(2), 2332858417706899. 10.1177/233285841 7706899

Doabler, C. T., Clarke, B., Kosty, D., Kurtz-Nelson, E., Fien, H., Smolkowski, K., & Baker, S. K. (2019). Examining the impact of group size on the treatment intensity of a tier 2 mathematics intervention within a systematic framework of replication. *Journal of Learning Disabilities, 52*(2), 168–180. 10.1177/0022219418789376

Doabler, C. T., Fien, H., Nelson-Walker, N. J., & Baker, S. K. (2012). Evaluating Three Elementary Mathematics Programs for Presence of Eight Research-Based Instructional Design Principles. *Learning Disability Quarterly, 35*(4), 200–211.

Dombrowski, S. C., J. McGill, R., Farmer, R. L., Kranzler, J. H., & Canivez, G. L. (2021). Beyond the rhetoric of evidence-based assessment: A framework for critical thinking in clinical practice. *School Psychology Review, 51*(6), 771–784. 10.1080/2372966X.2021.1960126

Duhon, G. J., Poncy, B. C., & Krawiec, C. F. (2022). Toward a more comprehensive evaluation of interventions: A dose-response curve analysis of an explicit timing intervention. *School Psychology, 51*(1), 84–94.

Farmer, R. L., Zaheer, I., & Duhon, G. J. (2021). Reducing low-value practices a functional-contextual consideration to aid in de-implementation efforts. *Canadian Journal of School Psychology, 36*(2), 153–165.

Francis, D. J., Fletcher, J. M., Stuebing, K. K., Lyon, G. R., Shaywitz, B. A., & Shaywitz, S. E. (2005). Psychometric approaches to the identification of LD: IQ and achievement scores are not sufficient. *Journal of Learning Disabilities, 38*(2), 98–108. 10.1177/00222194050380020101

Garet, M. S., Cronen, S., Eaton, M., Kurki, A., Ludwig, M., Jones, W., ... & Sztejnberg, L. (2008). The impact of two professional development interventions on early reading instruction and achievement. NCEE 2008-4030. *National Center for Education Evaluation and Regional Assistance.*

Garet, M. S., Heppen, J. B., Walters, K., Parkinson, J., Smith, T. M., Song, M., ... & Borman, G. D. (2016). Focusing on mathematical knowledge: The impact of content-intensive teacher professional development. NCEE 2016-4010. *National Center for Education Evaluation and Regional Assistance.*

Garet, M. S., Wayne, A. J., Stancavage, F., Taylor, J., Eaton, M., Walters, K., ... & Doolittle, F .(2011). Middle school mathematics professional development impact study: Findings after the second year of implementation. NCEE 2011-4024. *National Center for Education Evaluation and Regional Assistance.*

Hale, J., Alfonso, V., Berninger, V., Bracken, B., Christo, C., Clark, E., Cohen, M., Davis, A., Decker, S., Denckla, M., & Others. (2010). Critical issues in response-to-intervention, comprehensive evaluation, and specific learning disabilities identification and intervention: An expert white paper consensus. *Learning Disability Quarterly: Journal of the Division for Children with Learning Disabilities*, 33(3), 223–236. https://journals.sagepub.com/doi/abs/10.1177/0731 94871003300310?casa_token=Ux8yiPBVPfEAAAAA:_DjdARA_MXVmchhTYdi yc4TIkxjMPaMP4f8osvFGZAYqR-n9WVL46uqNE2BKI5GY60Rb7L_kHo_B

Hanushek, E. A. (2011). The economic value of higher teacher quality. *Economics of Education Review*, 30(3), 466–479. 10.1016/j.econedurev.2010.12.006

Haring, N. G., & Eaton, M. D. (1978). Systematic instructional procedures: An instructional hierarchy. *The Fourth R: Research in the Classroom.*

Hernandez-Nuhfer, M. P., Poncy, B. C., Duhon, G., Solomon, B. G., & Skinner, C. H. (2020). Factors influencing the effectiveness of interventions: An interaction of instructional set size and dose. *School Psychology Review*, 49(4), 386–398. 10.1080/2372966X.2020.1777832

January, S. A. A., & Klingbeil, D. A. (2020). Universal screening in grades K-2: A systematic review and meta-analysis of early reading curriculum-based measures. *Journal of School Psychology*, 82, 103–122.

Kane, M. (2013). The argument-based approach to validation. *School Psychology Review*, 42(4), 448–457. 10.1080/02796015.2013.12087465

Kilgus, S. P., Methe, S. A., Maggin, D. M., & Tomasula, J. L. (2014). Curriculum-based measurement of oral reading (R-CBM): A diagnostic test accuracy meta-analysis of evidence supporting use in universal screening. *Journal of School Psychology*, 52(4), 377–405

Kovaleski, J. F., VanDerHeyden, A. M., Runge, T. J., Zirkel, P. A., & Shapiro, E. S. (2022). *The RTI approach to evaluating learning disabilities.* Guilford Publications. https://play.google.com/store/books/details?id=XmKJEAAAQBAJ

Macmann, G. M., & Barnett, D. W. (1985). Discrepancy score analysis: A computer simulation of classification stability. *Journal of Psychoeducational Assessment*, 3(4), 363–375. 10.1177/073428298500300409

Messick, S. (1986). The once and future issues of validity: Assessing the meaning and consequences of measurement1. *ETS Research Report Series*, 1986(2), i–24. 10.1002/j.2330-8516.1986.tb00185.x

Miciak, J., & Fletcher, J. M. (2019). The Identification of Reading Disabilities, *Reading Development and Difficulties: Bridging the Gap between Research and Practice* (pp. 159–177).

Miciak, J., Fletcher, J. M., Stuebing, K. K., Vaughn, S., & Tolar, T. D. (2014). Patterns of cognitive strengths and weaknesses: Identification rates, agreement, and validity for learning disabilities identification. *School Psychology Quarterly*, 29(1), 21–37.

Miciak, J., Williams, J. L., Taylor, W. P., Cirino, P. T., Fletcher, J. M., & Vaughn, S. (2016). Do processing patterns of strengths and weaknesses predict differential treatment response?. *Journal of Educational Psychology*, *108*(6), 898–909.

Newell, K. W., Codding, R. S., & Fortune, T. W. (2020). Oral reading fluency as a screening tool with English learners: A systematic review. *Psychology in the Schools*, *57*(8), 1208–1239.

Shaw, S. R. (2021). Implementing evidence-based practices in school psychology: Excavation by de-implementing the disproved. *Canadian Journal of School Psychology*, *36*(2), 91–97. 10.1177/08295735211000513

Slavin, R. E., & Lake, C. (2008). Effective Programs in Elementary Mathematics: A Best-Evidence Synthesis. *Review of Educational Research*, *78*(3), 427–515.

Solomon, B. G., Poncy, B. C., Battista, C., & Campaña, K. V. (2020). A review of common rates of improvement when implementing whole-number operation math interventions. *School Psychology*, *35*(5), 353–362. 10.1037/spq0000360

Stuebing, K. K., Barth, A. E., Molfese, P. J., Weiss, B., & Fletcher, J. M. (2009). IQ is not strongly related to response to reading instruction: A meta-analytic interpretation. *Exceptional Children*, *76*(1), 31–51. 10.1177/001440290907600102

Travers, J. C. (2017). Evaluating claims to avoid pseudoscientific and unproven practices in special education. *Intervention in School and Clinic*, *52*(4), 195–203. 10.1177/1053451216659466

Reschly, A. L., & Coolong-Chaffin (2016). Contextual influences and response to intervention. In S. R. Jimerson, M. K. Burns, & A. M. VanDerHeyden (Eds.). *Handbook of response to intervention*. Springer.

VanDerHeyden, A. M., Broussard, C., & Burns, M. K. (2021). Classification agreement for gated screening in mathematics: Subskill mastery measurement and classwide intervention. *Assessment for Effective Intervention: Official Journal of the Council for Educational Diagnostic Services*, *46*(4), 270–280. 10.1177/1534508419882484

VanDerHeyden, A. M., Burns, M. K., & Bonifay, W. (2018). Is more screening better? The relationship between frequent screening, accurate decisions, and reading proficiency. *School Psychology Review*, *47*(1), 62–82. 10.17105/spr-2017-0017. v47-1

VanDerHeyden, A. M., & Codding, R. S. (2015). Practical effects of classwide mathematics intervention. *School Psychology Review*, *44*(2), 169–190. 10.17105/spr-13-0087.1

VanDerHeyden, A. M., Codding, R., & Solomon, B. G. (2022). Reliability of computer-based CBMs versus paper/pencil administration for fact and complex operations in mathematics. *Remedial and Special Education*. 10.1177/0741 9325221079851

VanDerHeyden, A. M., & Witt, J. C. (2005). Quantifying context in assessment: capturing the effect of base rates on teacher referral and a problem-solving model of identification. *School Psychology Review*, *34*(2), 161–183. 10.1080/02796015.2005.12086281

Watkins, M. W., & Canivez, G. L. (2022). Are There Cognitive Profiles Unique to Students With Learning Disabilities? A Latent Profile Analysis of Wechsler Intelligence Scale for Children–Fourth Edition Scores. *School Psychology Review*, *51*(5), 634–646.

8 Projective Drawing Techniques

*Nicholas F. Benson, Stefan C. Dombrowski,
and Michael I. Axelrod*

Projective assessment, or assessment techniques that rely on ambiguous stimuli to elicit responses revealing elements of an individual's personality or underlying psychopathology, has a long-standing history in clinical and school psychology. The practice started to flourish in the late 19th century and was used in schools in the 1950s and 1960s to identify children with various psychological disorders and label their condition (Anastasi, 1988; Mihura & Meyer, 2022, Peterson & Batsche, 1983). While the role of projective assessment in school psychology has declined over time, about one-third of current practitioners continue to engage in their use, most notably through projective drawing techniques (Benson et al., 2019). Projective drawing techniques, namely, Draw-A-Person (DAP), Kinetic Family Drawing (KFD), and House-Tree-Person (HTP), were cited by school psychologists as the most frequently used projective assessments. The purpose of this chapter is to critically examine claims underlying projective drawing techniques, one subset of projective assessment.

An underlying premise of projective techniques is that responses provided by the examinee are either unknown (i.e., unconscious) or unable to be communicated; otherwise, the examiner would ask the examinee about it directly (Rapaport et al., 1945–1946). The premise here is that the examinee "projects" useful information from their unconscious into the drawing itself. Ambiguity is viewed as a desirable property for projective techniques. The use of ambiguous stimuli in projective techniques is thought to provide a subtle, indirect approach to uncovering implicit (i.e., unconscious, automatic) psychological schemas (e.g., perceptions, cognitions, or behavioral styles) believed to underlie mental functioning and behavior. These implicit schemas are thought to operate automatically in high-ambiguity situations, and personal schemas (i.e., knowledge structures used to organize and interpret information) are believed to play a particularly notable role in how individual's respond to ambiguous stimuli in real-life situations. Implicit personal schemas "are outgrowths of experiences, incorporating ideas about sources of emotions

DOI: 10.4324/9781003266181-11

such as distress or about efficacy to regulate uncomfortable states, to cope with challenges, or to attain desired outcomes" (Teglasi, 2013, p. 14).

This chapter will examine five primary claims: 1) projective drawings can be administered, scored, and interpreted using standardized approaches, 2) projective drawings have strong evidence of reliability, 3) projective drawings have strong evidence of validity, 4) projective drawings are useful for diagnosis, and 5) projective drawings are useful for treatment planning.

Examining the Claims

Claim #1: Projective Drawings Can Be Administered, Scored, and Interpreted Using Standardized Approaches

Advocates for using projective drawings in child and adolescent assessment claim standardized approaches to administration, scoring, and interpretation exist. First, specific instructions may be provided to the examinee. For example, HTP uses an arranged sequence – the child is given a booklet and pencil, and then asked to draw a house, tree, person, and person of the opposite sex in that order. Second, structured scoring systems have been developed to systematize interpretation. For example, DAP has a quantitative scoring system to measure nonverbal features of intelligence. Finally, interpretative models exist to support inferences about underlying problems and diagnostic conceptualizations. For example, the KFD scoring system includes four broad categories for interpreting drawings – actions of the figures (e.g., cooperation, narcissism, and tension), physical characteristics (e.g., side of body parts relative to other figures, facial expressions), distance, barriers, and positions (e.g., direction each figure faces, objective between two figures), and styles (e.g., organization of figures on the page). The styles category is said to reflect emotional disturbance and psychopathology.

While there might be examples of standardization in administration, scoring, and interpretation of projective drawings, questions remain as to the veracity of these attempts to standardize projective drawing practices. Despite evidence that standardized administration procedures exist for project drawing assessments, there is considerable variability across assessment protocols with many providing little to no direction to examinees (Hunsley et al., 2015). For example, KFD requires the child to draw their family doing something together and DAP has the child simply draw a picture of a person. The nondirective nature of the instructions might influence children's drawings. Burkitt (2017) found that varying details when instructing children to draw pictures influenced their drawings. Regarding scoring systems, many proponents of projective drawings advocate using a nonstandardized scoring approach (Whitcomb, 2018). However, standardized scoring procedures exist but are not well supported.

Idiosyncratic scoring, inadequate norms, and the ignoring of important gender differences all plague projective drawing scoring systems (Groth-Marnat, 1997; Hensley et al., 2015; Whitcomb, 2018). Finally, scholars have noted the subjectivity associated with interpreting projective drawings. Although scoring schemes attempt to standardize interpretation, fair criticisms exist concerning interpretive practices made from biased judgments. For example, a descriptive study by Smith and Dumont (1995) found both experienced and novice psychologists' interpretations of DAP were representative of the illusory correlation (i.e., the perceiving a false relationship between a drawing and underlying psychological problems). They also discovered that many of the interpretations assumed an isomorphic relationship between the drawing and the person (e.g., lots of buckles and buttons mean dependency), despite research indicating specific features of a drawing fail to correlate with specific personality features. Other research has found clinician interpretations are frequently centered on intuitively based associations (e.g., small figure suggests poor self-confidence; Groth-Marnat, 1997).

Claim #2: Projective Drawings Have Strong Evidence of Reliability

Proponents of projective drawing techniques claim these assessment procedures are reliable. That is, projective drawings demonstrate adequate consistency across drawing components (i.e., internal consistency), raters (i.e., interrater reliability), and assessment administrations (i.e., test–retest reliability). Efforts to examine the reliability of projective techniques, including projective drawings, are challenging due to the proliferation of stimuli presentation options, directions for task completion, and scoring systems. Moreover, reliability is influenced by the wide range of examinee responses given projective drawings tend to be minimally structured.

Research investigating the internal consistency, interrater reliability, and test–retest reliability of children's projective drawing assessments has yielded mixed results. For example, interrater agreement with specific scoring systems (e.g., DAP: *Screening Procedure for Emotional Disturbance* [DAP: SPED]) has been reported to range from 75% to 95% indicating strong interrater reliability and there is moderate support for internal consistency with coefficients ranging from .58 to .78 (Lilienfeld et al., 2000; McGrath & Carroll, 2012; Whitcomb, 2018). However, research reviews have highlighted problems with the reliability of projective drawing assessments. Studies of interrater reliability have produced highly variable results, as reported coefficients range from .01 to 1.0, with the average interrater reliability at approximately .50 (Lilienfeld et al., 2000; McGrath & Carroll, 2012; Whitcomb, 2018). Research on test–retest reliability has also been variable, with reliability coefficients ranging from the .40 s to the .90 s (Whitcomb, 2018).

The claim that projective drawing assessments have reliability is problematic. Although research has demonstrated strong reliability, there is obvious variation across studies. This variation might be an artifact of many things including the population (e.g., age, gender, presence, and absence of psychopathology) or the clinician's experience scoring the projective drawing. Moreover, Whitcomb (2018) noted these reported reliability coefficients, when compared to other social/emotional assessment types (e.g., behavior rating scales), indicate strong inconsistency and that the data are enough to conclude "that it is likely children will produce qualitatively different drawings from one occasion to another" (p. 254). Finally, there are several features and unresolved issues associated with projective drawings used with children that question their reliability. For example, it is largely unknown whether projective drawings are state- or trait-dependent measures. Cummings (1980) suggested projective drawings used with children may, in fact, assess feelings, perceptions, and affect at a specific point in time rather than capture long-standing personality characteristics.

Claim #3: Projective Drawings Have Strong Evidence of Validity

Proponents of projective drawings claim these assessment procedures validly identify characteristics of psychopathology and underlying causes of problems, thus making them useful for diagnosis. Efforts to examine the validity of projective drawing assessments with children are challenging for the same reasons as noted for reliability. In addition, clinician and researcher interpretations of projective drawings are seemingly difficult to falsify (i.e., experimentally determined as false; Lilienfeld et al., 2000). For example, Ballús et al. (2023) hypothesized that omissions or distortions (e.g., missing feet, large head) of body parts in children's projective drawings would be predictive of the presence of emotional problems. Studying a sample of children receiving treatment for abuse or neglect, the researchers concluded that most drawings depicted emotional indicators common to abuse or neglect and confirmed emotional problems. In addition to problems existing with the sample (i.e., children with histories of abuse or neglect and likely emotional problems), the researchers speculated that those features found in the children's drawings were indicative of psychopathology despite no systematic evaluation to test this predictive hypothesis. Foley and Mullis (2008) also asserted that features of children's drawings could be used to identify problems. For example, they contended that the shading of lines (i.e., heavy or light) was associated with aggression and anxiety, citing interpretive manuals rather than experimental studies to support their claims.

In addition to the challenges in falsifying interpretive claims, evidence supporting the validity of projective drawings is minimal at best. Reviews investigating the psychometric properties of projective drawings with children and adolescents have concluded the assessments have poor levels of validity (Lilienfeld et al., 2000, Hensley et al., 2015; McGrath & Carroll, 2012; Miller & Nickerson, 2006; Whitcomb, 2018). This is particularly evident when single indicators (e.g., missing feet, large hands, line shading, and figure size) are used to make inferences about psychopathology. For example, Joiner et al. (1996) studied the relationship between three commonly used single indicators of emotional distress used to interpret children's drawings (i.e., size, detail, and line heaviness) and self-report measures of anxiety and depression in a sample of psychiatric inpatient children. The researchers found that, despite high interrater reliability, the drawings were not significantly correlated with self-reported anxiety or depression. These results are consistent with Whitcomb's (2018) assessment of the literature, noting that few studies exist demonstrating a correlation between projective drawing indicators and other behavioral, emotional, and social measures (e.g., behavior rating scales).

Examining projective drawings using specific scoring schemes yields similar findings. For example, Wrightson and Saklofske (2000) found that scores from the DAP:SPED failed to discriminate between groups of students with mild versus significant behavior problems. DAP:SPED scores differentiated between students with and without behavior problems but the researchers cautioned interpreting these results as validating the DAP:SPED. Mean DAP:SPED global scores for all three groups were in the average range, whereas mean scores from the *Child Behavior Checklist* and *Devereux Behavior Rating Scale* were in the average range for students without behavior problems and in the clinical range for students with behavior problems. The researchers concluded the DAP:SPED provided no additional information that could otherwise be ascertained from the rating scales and, in fact, might be plagued by too many false negatives (i.e., indicating a serious behavior problem does not exist when it actually does exist). Similar research has been conducted using projective drawing scoring schemes and other relevant constructs. Troncone et al. (2021) found scores from the *Quantitative Scoring System from the DAP* (DAP:QSS) failed to correlate with measures of children's intellectual functioning despite the DAP:QSS being designed to measure intellectual level without the influence of linguistic variables (see Naglieri, 1988). The researchers also found DAP:QSS scores were also not correlated with academic achievement and questioned the overall psychometric properties of the assessment.

Wrightson and Saklofske's (2000) conclusion, in many ways, addressed the concern about the incremental validity of projective drawings with children and adolescents. Incremental validity refers to the extent to which an assessment offers unique information about a construct relative to information provided by other assessments purported to measure the same construct. Proponents of projective assessments encourage practitioners to use them within the context of a larger evaluation asserting they add an additional source of information and, thus, enhancing the incremental validity of the information obtained (Koppitz, 1983). However, very few studies have examined the incremental validity of children's projective drawings and those that have been plagued by methodological problems (e.g., using only some items from teacher ratings). In their comprehensive review, Lilienfeld et al. (2000) noted "there is no convincing evidence that human figure drawings possess incremental validity above and beyond other readily available demographic or psychometric data" (p. 51).

Claim #4: Projective Drawings Are Useful for Diagnosis

Conclusions drawn from the research on the psychometric properties of children's projective drawings suggest the assessment technique is problematic as a diagnostic tool. Studies demonstrating modest reliability coefficients and poor validity, especially incremental validity, question the usefulness of projective drawings as part of a larger battery of tests when making diagnostic decisions. Studies attempting to use projective drawing scoring schemes (e.g., DAP:SPED) to differentiate clinical and normal samples of children to establish a system's utility in diagnostic decision-making often detect statistically significant mean differences but the means of both groups are reported to be within the average range (e.g., Naglieri & Pfeiffer, 1992; Wrightson & Saklofske, 2000). Although the clinical and non-clinical groups in these studies differed statistically, the difference's practical significance is questionable. Furthermore, these findings suggest low sensitivity (i.e., a test's ability to identify an individual with a disorder) and high false positive and negative rates (see Troncone et al., 2021). In addition, research on interpretive frameworks claiming specific characteristics within a drawing could differentiate between different groups of children has yielded contradictory findings. In reviewing the relevant research, Cummings (1986) found studies demonstrating children with and without emotional problems were distinguished by certain style indicators (e.g., emphasis on physical properties, outdoor pictures) but some studies indicated children with emotional problems had more style indicators while other studies revealed children without emotional problems had more style indicators. Finally, factors other than psychopathology are likely responsible for differentiated responses to drawing prompts. For example, artistic ability is a potential extraneous or confounding variable in research investigating the relationship between projective drawings and features of psychopathology (Lilienfeld et al., 2000).

The utility of projective drawings and their scoring systems diagnostic tool is weak given the existing evidence. Comprehensive reviews of the research regularly caution practitioners about the limitations of using projective drawings for diagnosis or, perhaps more relevant to school psychologists, the determination of eligibility for special education (Hunsley et al., 2015; Lilienfeld et al., 2000, Whitcomb, 2018). Moreover, school psychology scholars have concluded that projective drawings are not needed in the assessment of children and adolescent psychopathology (see Miller & Nickerson, 2006). School psychologists have available to them an array of assessment tools with strong psychometric properties (e.g., behavior rating scales) that, when used with other evaluation techniques (e.g., interviews, observations), can provide useful diagnostic information.

Proponents of projective drawing techniques contend their predictive value has as much to do with the examiner's qualifications (e.g., knowledge, experience, and skills) than the assessment's psychometric properties (Koppitz, 1983). Said differently, claims about the validity of children's projective drawings rest on the importance of nuanced interpretations and clinical judgment. Yet, research fails to support this assertion (see Garb, 1989, 1998; Lilienfeld et al., 2000). For example, Levenberg's (1975) often-cited study found doctoral-level clinicians, predoctoral interns, and hospital secretaries did not differ in overall level of diagnostic accuracy when interpreting KFDs to differentiate between children with and without psychopathology. Most concerning, the KFD expert's hit rate was significantly less accurate than the overall mean (47% vs. 65%) and markedly lower than any of the experimental groups identifying children with psychopathology. In reviewing the literature, Cummings (1986) questioned whether clinical judgment could be robust enough to prevent large numbers of false positives and whether clinicians could properly avoid confirming pre-established hypotheses when interpreting children's drawings.

Claim #5: Projective Drawings Are Useful for Intervention

Proponents claim that projective drawings are useful for intervention. For example, Foley and Mullis (2008) suggest children's projective drawings could be employed in schools to design interventions. Others have made similar assertions about the treatment utility of the projective drawings of children and adolescents. Using drawings to assess for psychopathology (e.g., anxiety, depression), sexual abuse, impulsiveness, and problems in interpersonal relationships through various interpretive approaches has the potential to inform treatment. However, there is scant evidence indicating projective drawings are useful for treatment planning. Moreover, published research regarding the effectiveness with which school psychologists can use projective drawings to improve intervention outcomes for students is absent. Finally, all projective assessments require a high level of inference and other evaluation approaches are available that have better psychometric properties and offer a greater link between assessment and intervention (e.g., functional behavior assessment).

Some scholars assert that projective techniques could be useful for establishing rapport with students, observing students, and facilitating discussions with students about important topics (see Foley and Mullis, 2008; Miller & Nickerson, 2006). Others have echoed similar sentiments, suggesting projective drawings might be beneficial when used under certain circumstances. For example, Stark (1990) suggested projective techniques may be useful with children with depression who are apprehensive to openly disclose what they are thinking and feeling, and Karp (1997) provided a case study illustrating the use of projective drawings as a communication tool between a therapist and child. Such practices in a therapeutic context might have some value; however, practitioners are cautioned to avoid jumping to conclusions or generating hypotheses from drawings. Finally, some have recommended utilizing projective drawing procedures, especially the KFD, within clinical interview frameworks to support communication about family dynamics (Lee et al., 2017) or understand discrepant assessment findings to identify treatment targets (Achenbach & Rescorla, 2004), although research supporting these applications does not exist.

Summary and Conclusion

The sustained use of projective drawings with children and adolescents is intriguing given the general lack of evidence supporting most score interpretations and uses. Some who promote or utilize unsupported practices may remain unaware of the evidence base. However, there are other factors that influence instrument selection. Could the enduring use of projective techniques be related to their intuitive appeal and perhaps an unsophisticated understanding of the research process (Zachar & Leong, 2000)? Could it also be related to how such practices are promoted in psychology which may well have greater reach than scientific journals (see Dombrowski et al., 2022). The interplay of commercial promotion, with its concomitant conflicts of interest, and evidence-based practices sometimes results in conflicting priorities resulting in allegiance networks, group identity conflicts, and ideological capture (see Prataknis, 1995; Herbert et al., 2000 for an example of a ubiquitous practice that uses tactics of pseudoscientific marketing; see Dombrowski et al., 2022 for a more detailed discussion of why low-value practices persist despite evidence against those practices).

In contexts that involve important issues such as psychological distress, physical health, and social justice, Meehl (1973) contended that allowing others to "persist in egregious mistakes ... is not only foolish, it is downright immoral" (p. 299). Indeed, basing high-stakes decisions on invalid uses of projective drawings can result in harm. Moreover, using projective techniques, including drawings, for detecting serious crimes against children (e.g., child sexual abuse) despite no established validity for this purpose is disturbing (see Lilienfeld et al., 2000).

Appeals to the continued use of projective techniques based on "clinicians' faith in the incremental validity of implicit measures over self-report measures" and unverified beliefs of what "gifted clinicians" can accomplish (McGrath & Carroll, 2012, p. 342) can be viewed as warning signs of hype and pseudoscience (Farmer et al., 2022). Likewise, arguments against constraining the use of projective techniques, including and especially children's drawings, based on perceived errors of omission and commission in reviews of validity evidence (e.g., Hibbard, 2003) may suggest a perspective antithetical to evidence-based practice. Evidence-based practice involves the conscientious, explicit, and circumspect use of current best evidence (i.e., research findings and clinical expertise; American Psychological Association, Presidential Task Force on Evidence-Based Practice, 2006). While an absence of evidence is not evidence that a practice is invalid, the burden of proof lies with those who promote practices.

Decades-old admonitions (e.g., Knoff, 1993; Lilienfeld et al., 2000) for practitioners and trainers to discontinue the use and instruction of projective techniques largely continue to ring true. Relative to adults, there is much less evidence supporting their with children. Moreover, there is a paucity of evidence supporting their use in school settings for purposes such as determining eligibility for special education or informing the design of interventions. There may be reasonable situations in which a school psychologist asks a student to do a drawing. For example, the drawing could be a useful starting point to have a conversation. In addition, having students draw may be useful within a larger therapeutic context such as a student with a debilitating fear of dogs being encouraged to draw a dog as part of exposure therapy exercises. However, there are plenty of reasons to be skeptical when a drawing's purpose involves assessing referral concerns by having the student project unconscious information onto a page. It is possible that future drawing techniques may be constructed in a way that they are worth using for school psychologists, and we have to remain open to that possibility. Simultaneously, we must remain skeptical as the claims made by the authors of projective techniques have not lived up to the evidence base.

References

American Educational Research Association, American Psychological Association, & National Council on Measurement in Education (2014). Standards for educational and psychological testing (4th ed.). Authors.

American Psychological Association, Presidential Task Force on Evidence-Based Practice (2006). Evidence-based practice in psychology. American Psychologist, *61*, 271–285.

Achenbach, T. M., & Rescorla, L. (2004). Practical applications of the Achenbach System of Empirically Based Assessment (ASEBA) for ages 1.5 to 90+ years [Paper presentation]. The International Test Users' Conference. https://research.acer.edu.au/research_conferenceITU_2004/2

Anastasi, A. (1988). Psychological testing (6th ed.). Macmillan.

Ballüs, E., Comelles, C., Pasto, T., & Benedico, P. (2023). Children's drawings as a projective tool to explore and prevent experiences of mistreatment and/or sexual abuse. Frontiers in Psychology, *14*, 1002864.

Benson, N. F., Floyd, R. G., Kranzler, J. H., Eckert, T. L., Fefer, S. A., & Morgan, G. B. (2019). Test use and assessment practices of school psychologists in the United States: Findings from the 2017 National Survey. Journal of School Psychology, *72*, 29–48.

Burkitt, E. (2017). The effects of task explicitness to communicate on the expressiveness of children's drawings of different topics. Educational Psychology, *37*, 219–236.

Cummings, J. A. (1980). *An evaluation of objective scoring systems for the Kinetic Family Drawings* (Publication No. 41(6)) [Doctoral dissertation, University of Georgia].

Cummings, J. A. (1986). Projective drawings. In H. Knoff (Ed.), The assessment of child and adolescent personality (pp. 199–244). Guilford.

Dombrowski, S. C., J. McGill, R., Farmer, R. L., Kranzler, J. H., & Canivez, G. L. (2021). Beyond the rhetoric of evidence-based assessment: A framework for critical thinking in clinical practice. School Psychology Review, 1–14.

Farmer, R. L., McGill, R. J., Lockwood, A. B., Dombrowski, S. C., Canivez, G. L., & Zaheer, I. (2022). Warning signs of hype in school-based assessment: Implications for training and pedagogy. School Psychology Training & Pedagogy, *39*(1). [https://psyarxiv.com/ypcv7]

Foley, Y. C., & Mullis, F. (2008). Interpreting children's human figure drawings: Basic guidelines for school counselors. GSCA Journal, *1*, 28–37.

Garb, H. N. (1998). Studying the clinician: Judgment research and psychological assessment. Washington, DC: American Psychological Association.

Garb, H. N. (1989). Clinical judgment, clinical training, and professional experience. Psychological Bulletin, *105*, 387–396.

Groth-Marnat, G. (1997). Handbook of psychological assessment (Third Edition). Wiley.

Herbert, J. D., Lilienfeld, S. O., Lohr, J. M., Montgomery, R. W., O'Donohue, W. T., Rosen, G. M., & Tolin, D. F. (2000). Science and pseudoscience in the development of eye movement desensitization and reprocessing: Implications for clinical psychology. Clinical Psychology Review, *20*(8), 945–971.

Hibbard, S. (2003). A critique of Lilienfeld et al.'s (2000) "The scientific status of projective techniques." Journal of Personality Assessment, *80*(3), 260–271.

Hunsley, J., Lee, C. M., Wood, J. M., & Taylor, W. (2015). Controversial and questionable assessment techniques. In S. O. Lilienfeld, S. J. Lynn, & J. M. Lohr (Eds.), Science and pseudoscience in clinical psychology (pp. 42–82). Guilford.

Joiner, T. E., Schmidt, K. L., & Barnett, J. (1996). Size, detail, and line heaviness in children's drawings as correlates of emotional distress: (More) negative evidence. Journal of Personality Assessment, *67*, 127–141.

Karp, M. R. (1997). Symbolic participation: The role of projective drawings in a case of child abuse. Psychoanalytic Study of the Child, *52*, 260–300.

Knoff, Howard M. (1993). The utility of human figure drawings in personality and intellectual assessment: Why ask why? School Psychology Quarterly, 8, 191–196.

Koppitz, E. M. (1983). Projective drawings with children and adolescents. School Psychology Review, *12*, 421–427.

Lee, B. M., Lim, B. H., & Chia, K. H. (2017). Kinetic family drawing interview questionnaire (KFD-IQ): A tool to learn about the family unit from a drawer's perspective. European Journal of Special Education Research, *2*, 102–119.

Levenberg, S. B. (1975). Professional training, psychodiagnostics skill, and kinetic family drawings. Journal of Personality Assessment, *39*, 389–393.

Lilienfeld, S. O., Wood, J. M., & Garb, H. N. (2000). The scientific status of projective techniques. Psychological Science in the Public Interest, *1*, 27–66.

McGrath, R. E., & Carroll, E. J. (2012). The current *status* of "projective" "tests". In H. Cooper (Ed.), APA handbook of research methods in psychology: Vol 1. Foundations, planning, measures, and psychometrics (pp. 329–348). American Psychological Association.

Meehl, P. E., (1973). Why I do not attend case conferences. In P. E. Meehl (Ed.), Psychodiagnosis: Selected papers (pp. 225–302). University of Minnesota Press.

Mihura, J. L., & Meyer, G. J. (2022). The Rorschach Performance Assessment System (R-PAS) in multimethod assessment [chapter-in-press]. In J. L. Mihura (Ed.), The Oxford handbook of personality and psychopathology assessment. Oxford.

Miller, D. N., & Nickerson, A. B. (2006). Projective assessment and school psychology: Contemporary validity issues and implications for practice. The California School Psychologist, *11*, 73–84.

Naglieri, J. A. (1988). Draw-a-person: A quantitative scoring system. San Antonio, TX: The Psychological Corporation.

Naglieri, J. A., & Pfeiffer, S. I. (1992). Performance of disruptive behavior-disordered and normal samples on the Draw-A-Person: Screening procedure for emotional disturbance. Psychological Assessment, *4*, 156–159.

Peterson, D. W., & Batsche, G. M. (1983). School psychology and projective assessment: A growing incompatibility. School Psychology Review, *12*, 440–445.

Pratkanis, A. R. (1995). How to sell a pseudoscience. The Skeptical Inquirer, *19*, 19–25.

Rapaport, D., Gill, M., & Schafer, R. (1945–1946). Diagnostic psychological testing (Vols 1–2). Yearbook Publishers.

Smith, D., & Dumont, F. (1995). A cautionary study: Unwarranted interpretation of the Draw-A-Person test. Professional Psychology: Research and Practice, *26*, 298–303.

Stark, K. D. (1990). Childhood depression: School-based intervention. New York: Guilford.

Teglasi, H. (2013). The scientific status of projective techniques as performance measures of personality. In D. H. Saklofske, C. R. Reynolds, & V. L. Schwean (Eds.), The Oxford handbook of child psychological assessment. (pp. 113–128). Oxford University Press.

Troncone, A., Chianese, A., Di Leva, A., Grasso, M., & Cascella, C. (2021). Validity of the Draw A Person: A Quantitative Scoring System (DAP:QSS) for clinically evaluating intelligence. Child Psychiatry & Human Development, *52*, 728–738.

Whitcomb, S. A. (2018). Behavioral, social, and emotional assessment of children and adolescents (Fifth Edition). Routledge.

Wrightson, L., & Saklofske, D. H. (2000). Validity and reliability of the draw a person: Screening procedure for emotional disturbance with adolescent students. Canadian Journal of School Psychology, *16*, 95–102.

Zachar, P., & Leong, F. T. (2000). A 10-year longitudinal study of scientists and practitioner interests in psychology: Assessing the Boulder model. Professional Psychology: Research and Practice, *31*, 575–580.

Part IV

Instruction and Intervention

9 Academic Instruction

Chad E. L. Kinney, John C. Begeny, and Rahma M. Hida

In this chapter, we explore beliefs and claims often regarded as unfounded in academic instruction in education. We examine where they come from, why they are problematic, what supports persistent belief in them, and how we might reduce their influence on academic instruction. Additionally, we provide some perspectives and suggestions aimed to offer (a) a healthy critique of pseudoscience as a concept and (b) some non-judgmental approaches to enhance the evaluation of and critical thinking about instructional methods.

Unfounded beliefs are "beliefs that are not supported by scientific evidence" (Caroti et al., 2022, p. 962). Pseudoscience – a category of unfounded beliefs – is a set of ideas, theories, or practices mistakenly perceived to be supported by the scientific method. For centuries, the influence of pseudoscience on global society has ranged from undeniably destructive (e.g., scientific racism) to arguably benign (e.g., astrology). In modern times, unfounded beliefs among educators have been high and steady over time, including over the past decade (Newton & Salvi, 2020; Torrijos-Muelas et al., 2021). Because this chapter pertains to academic instruction, we will limit our focus mainly to the pseudoscientific area called *neuromyths*.

Neuromyths are commonly held unfounded beliefs about brain functioning that are typically based on misunderstandings, bad interpretations, or distortions of neuroscientific research (Organisation for Economic Co-operation and Development [OCED], 2007). Neuromyths are relevant to education and academic instruction because they appeal to our interests in how the brain learns and are confused with evidence-based neuroscience (Grospietsch & Mayer, 2020).

Examining the Claims

The Prevalence of Neuromyths in Education

Across many countries, including the United States, neuromyths have been supported by a high percentage of educators (Dekker et al., 2012;

DOI: 10.4324/9781003266181-13

Ferrero et al., 2016; Grospietsch & Mayer, 2020; Newton & Miah, 2017; Newton & Salvi, 2020; Torrijos-Muelas et al., 2021; van Dijk & Lane, 2018). In the United Kingdom, Howard-Jones et al.'s (2009) survey found that over half of teachers-in-training agreed with a substantial number of neuromyths. Similar studies that followed also documented a high prevalence of educator support for neuromyths in China (Pei et al., 2015), Greece (Deligiannidi & Howard-Jones, 2015), Latin America (Gleichgerrcht et al., 2015), the Netherlands (Dekker et al., 2012), Portugal (Rato et al., 2013), Spain (Fuentes & Risso, 2015), and Turkey (Karakus et al., 2015).

Nearly a third of the articles in Torrijos-Muelas et al.'s (2021) systematic review of research on neuromyths in education relied on responses from pre-service educators-in-training. Some might reasonably contend that once these teachers-in-training complete their university coursework and gain teaching experience, their pseudoscientific beliefs will diminish. However, research findings do not support that contention. High percentages of in-service educators, educational leaders, and higher education faculty hold various pseudoscientific beliefs. For example, over 50% of higher education faculty supported (or did not dispute) pseudo-scientific claims related to education (e.g., learning styles) (Newton & Miah, 2017; van Dijk & Lane, 2018).

Learning Styles as a Neuromyth Example

Learning styles theory posits that learners can be categorized into one or more "styles" (e.g., visual, auditory, kinesthetic, and reading/writing) and can demonstrate improved learning when taught according to their learning style (Newton & Salvi, 2020). Repeated testing of this theory has generally yielded no supportive evidence (e.g., Rohrer & Pashler, 2012; Willingham et al., 2015); yet reported support for learning styles remains widespread among educators. In fact, learning styles theory is perhaps the most commonly accepted neuromyth (e.g., Lethaby & Harries, 2016; Newton & Salvi, 2020; Rousseau, 2021; Torrijos-Muelas et al., 2021).

Several studies have examined the prevalence of educators' beliefs in learning styles. Furey (2020) found that 29 states within the United States included learning styles theory in government-distributed test-preparation materials for teaching certification exams. A study in the United Kingdom found that 76% of schoolteachers reported using learning styles and linked their use to benefits for their students (Simmonds, 2014). Also, in the first part of Newton and Miah's (2017) survey of 114 higher education academics in the United Kingdom, about 58% of participants generally believed in the use of learning styles, and 33% of participants reported using the theory in practice. In the second part of Newton and Miah's

(2017) survey, the same participants received a research-based refutation of learning styles; subsequently, 32% of participants said they would continue applying the theory despite the lack of evidence to support it – thereby underscoring ineffective attempts within education to remove debunked neuromyths such as learning styles.

Other Common Neuromyth Examples

Research suggests that over 80% of educators support claims such as (a) short bouts of coordination exercises can improve integration of left and right hemispheric brain function (e.g., with brain gym activities), (b) differences between learners may be attributed to their brain hemispheric dominance (e.g., left brain vs. right brain dominance), and (c) the brain is like a hard drive that stores information in specific locations (Dekker et al., 2012; Lethaby & Harries, 2016; Grospietsch & Mayer, 2019). Similarly, one survey study (Macdonald et al., 2017) found that 55% of educators and 59% of the general public indicated support for the claim that classical music increases students' reasoning ability (i.e., the Mozart Effect).

A claim commonly known to special educators is that non-verbal people with autism are emotionally and cognitively neurotypical, but trapped within their own bodies. Moreover, to unlock their ability to learn and express themselves, they need facilitated communication. Facilitated communication involves a learner's dependence upon a trained professional to guide their selection of keys on a communication device, but scientific evidence has not supported that non-verbal autistic people engage in complex verbal expressions independent from the trained professional guiding their communication. Though scientific consensus was achieved about facilitated communication's ineffectiveness (Hemsley et al., 2018), the promotion of facilitated communication persists in academic and institutional settings to this day (Beals, 2022).

Reasons for Believing in Education-Based Neuromyths

Though unscientific beliefs about the brain and learning have existed for centuries, Dekker et al. (2012) noted a widespread interest among educators in applying neuroscientific research to students in the classroom since the 1990s "Decade of the Brain" in the United States. Pasquinelli (2012) describes how distortions and misinterpretations of neuroscientific research have passed through popular media to interested laypeople and thus perpetuate the existence of neuromyths. Furthermore, information and advertisements available through television, science magazines, or the Internet have been implicated in their contribution to neuromyths spreading throughout education settings (van Dijk & Lane, 2018;

Ferrero et al, 2016; Simmonds, 2014). In addition, pseudoscientific practices related to academic instruction have been promoted in professional development workshops, conferences, and educational materials for teachers (Busso & Pollack, 2015; Lethaby & Harries, 2016).

Pasquinelli (2012) also discussed how some neuromyths in education may have begun as peer-reviewed research, but later the research failed to be replicated by subsequent experiments and the ideas then became neuromyths as the public continued to adhere to outdated or debunked research. Examples of this are the Mozart effect and the learning styles theory. Further, the illusory effect (i.e., the finding that repeated information is often perceived as more truthful than new information) may also explain why neuromyths persist despite being debunked or lacking in evidence. For example, despite peer-reviewed articles exposing substantial methodological flaws in meta-analyses that support learning styles (e.g., Kavale & LeFever, 2007), studies highlighting learning styles have been cited far more often than articles debunking them (Newton & Salvi, 2020).

Another reason neuromyths survive may be that it can be difficult to distinguish between neuroscience and neuromyth (Dekker et al., 2012; Grospietsch & Mayer, 2020). An accurate understanding of neuroscientific methodology and terminology from which neuromyths spawn could require years of dedicated study (Pasquinelli, 2012). Moreover, some neuromyths have been identified to have a partial basis in scientific evidence or a "kernel of truth" that may seem to support them (Grospietsch & Mayer, 2019). For example, the learning styles theory is maintained by students' self-reported *preferences* for receiving information in a specific modality (Grospietsch & Mayer, 2020) and by research findings showing that different modes of information are processed in different parts of the brain (Dekker et al., 2012).

The Dangers of Believing in Neuromyths

A quick Google search will yield many organizations and individuals that perpetuate neuromyths by providing supportive information or by generating income from selling neuromyth-based materials and trainings. Such providers are often more than willing to supply the interested consumer with oodles of descriptive research, pilot studies, or anecdotal reports demonstrating their method's success. Naturally, some consumers will earnestly testify on the method's behalf, given their own experiences. In the case of guiding instructional practices based on learning styles theory, some students and parents may even find it problematic if the instructor or institution does *not* guide instruction with the student's learning styles in mind, which could affect how they rate instructors or institutions of learning on websites or evaluations.

Newton and Miah (2017) argued that instructional frameworks that rely on neuromyths are conceptually flawed, undermine the credibility of education, and waste valuable time, energy, and/or money that could be better spent on more effective, evidence-based instructional practices. Using conceptually flawed and non-empirically supported instructional strategies contradict the mission of maximizing students' learning and well-being. Moreover, if a neuromyth persists despite scientific evidence debunking it, what does that say about the credibility of an educational system? By allowing neuromyths to easily influence instructional practices, educational systems diminish the importance of science and verifiable evidence as mechanisms for achieving the highest possible impact on students' learning. Given significant inequities in education, any decline in evidence-based practice also diminishes advancements in equitable education. One striking example of the ways in which the application of neuromyths can contribute to wasting valuable time, energy, and money can be seen in state-level funding or policy making. In the case of widespread belief in the Mozart effect, Florida passed a bill in 1998 mandating daycare centers to play classical music to children, and the governor of Georgia at that time requested $105,000 from the state legislature to distribute classical music CDs to newborns (Pasquinelli, 2012).

Additional arguments for the problematic nature of neuromyths may be specific to the individual neuromyth. For example, when learners assume they cannot perform well if an instructional modality does not match their perceived learning style, they could become demotivated to continue learning, resulting in a self-fulfilling prophecy (Newton & Salvi, 2020). Also, if students have unrealistic expectations regarding how much time and energy an instructor needs to devote to accommodate their learning style, that might unfairly impact ratings of their instructor. More importantly, if a student did find their learning style was always accommodated by educators in the classroom, that might leave them unprepared to learn outside of the classroom when it is not feasible for on-the-job training to cater to personal learning preferences.

No matter how intellectually gifted or scientifically educated, a single human can only know a relatively tiny amount of all the world's knowledge. Thus, we believe it would also be dangerous to suggest that educators should halt their creativity and innovation and stop attempting new instructional strategies that are not yet thoroughly researched (i.e., an extreme reaction in the name of avoiding neuromyths). If a strategy is ethical, sound in principle, and informed by credible scientific evidence, there may be good reason for educators to implement those practices. Ideally, educators would also be involved with the systematic evaluation of any new strategies they try. However, if an instructional theory or strategy is scientifically determined to be ineffective, educators should abandon its practice.

What Supports Persistent Belief in Neuromyths?

Several psychological and cognitive factors may maintain our persistent belief in neuromyths. Processing information in the age of the Internet may be especially challenging in light of our exposure to constant floods of information and disinformation. Critical consumption of large amounts of complex data is difficult due to the limits of our cognitive resources, time, and knowledge; therefore, all individuals tend to use cognitive heuristics for credibility judgments. For example, people may be more likely to trust the judgments of friends and family over scientific findings (Eiser et al., 2009).

Another factor that may contribute to the maintenance of neuromyths, described as the anecdotal fallacy, is the tendency to use personal experience rather than evidence to support an argument. This may explain why educators who continued to use learning styles theory, despite contradicting evidence, rationalized their practice by citing their own positive personal experiences (e.g., Blanchette Sarrasin et al., 2019; Menz et al., 2021; Newton & Miah, 2017). Another relevant factor for the perpetuation of neuromyths is confirmation bias – the search for positive evidence that confirms our existing beliefs rather than information that disproves our views. Causal illusion – when people attribute a causal connection between two unrelated events – may also contribute to unfounded beliefs (Matute et al., 2015; Rousseau, 2021).

Increased scientific investigation of such biases may be useful for reliably describing general response patterns that can help us get closer to interventions that successfully dispel unfounded beliefs in general (including those about academic instruction). To avoid the circular reasoning of explaining away pseudoscientific instructional practices as "*caused* by cognitive biases," it is important that more research examines the social, cultural, and environmental conditions that evoke and maintain unfounded beliefs and biases. As suggested below, special training for educators may help reduce persistent beliefs in neuromyths.

What Can Be Done to Reduce the Influence of Neuromyths?

Rousseau (2021) published a recent review of research on interventions that aimed to dispel neuromyths, and these interventions primarily focused on providing refutations through books, articles, or lectures – sometimes provided in a university course. Refutation of neuromyths has been implemented by informing study participants why a particular neuromyth is false or providing research literature that debunks the pseudoscience (e.g., Newton & Miah, 2017). Refutation has also consisted of a single day of training on topics such as critical thinking, belief versus knowledge, and pseudoscience (Caroti et al., 2022), or even offering an entire university course on skepticism (e.g., Kane et al., 2010). Refutation has also come in the form of teaching students to avoid following an incorrect rule about causation by considering or testing information that would refute or disconfirm that rule (Barberia et al., 2018). Lastly, refutation research may involve having study participants write their own refutations and personal reflections on debunked neuromyths as part of the curriculum of a college course for teachers. For example, Grospietsch and Mayer (2018) used such methods and found dramatic reductions in student self-reports of endorsing multiple neuromyths (e.g., endorsement for providing instruction based on learning styles dropped from 95% to 38%).

Rousseau (2021) suggested that refutation-based interventions that rely on rational thinking, combined with emphasizing the use of alternative evidence-based instructional practices (suggested by Newton & Salvi, 2020), may fail to completely dispel neuromyths in education because both methods rest upon a foundation of an authoritative one-way dialogue between "expert" (scientist) and "student" (educator). Instead, having a bi-directional, non-condescending, and frequent dialog between researchers and educators – including collaborative research among them – may be more effective. These suggestions, however, require additional research.

University training for pre-service educators may also have a meaningful impact on the application of neuromyths in academic instruction. This may involve directly teaching skills related to critical thinking and consuming research (e.g., Kane et al., 2010), or it may involve a deeper assessment of what is included in students' curricula to become a professional educator. Blanchette Sarrasin et al. (2019) showed that 55% of participants' belief in learning styles was influenced by their university training. Additionally, some studies have found pre-service educators' general training in evidence-based instructional practices to be quite low (e.g., Vollmer et al., 2019). The multitude of complex influences on teacher education programs is beyond the scope of this chapter. However, ensuring that pre-service and in-service teachers receive sufficient curricular content and applied experiences that help them distinguish science from pseudoscience, may help to reduce pseudoscientific practices in classrooms.

Additional Considerations and Recommendations

Educational programs that lack scientific evidence for their effectiveness are far more common than programs that do have evidence of effectiveness (Gonzalez, 2018; Richardson, 2018); and some programs with evidence of effectiveness may be too unrealistic to implement in school-based settings (Gonzalez, 2018). Thus, we want to emphasize that (a) educators' instructional practices should be influenced by programs that have at least some scientifically valid evidence of being effective; (b) if such programs are not available or feasible for use in a respective context, appropriate and applied methods should be employed to evaluate programs in use that do not have scientific evidence; (c) instructional programs, methods, or theories that have been debunked through valid scientific inquiry should not be used; and (d) lack of empirical evidence for effectiveness does not automatically equate to using pseudoscientific practices, but it remains problematic to continue using instructional practices that lack evidence for effectiveness.

It is also important to critically consider the overarching concept of pseudoscience. For example, reports of scientific findings in education and psychology predominantly reflect countries in North America and Western Europe (Begeny et al., 2018; Thalmayer et al., 2021), possibly influencing what is prematurely dismissed as "pseudoscience." Scientific understanding is limited when participants living in locations that hold most of the world's population are excluded. Connected to this issue, academic neocolonialism (or academic imperialism) greatly influences scientific understanding (Alatas, 2003), and consumers of science must understand the influence of this form of neocolonialism when considering the evidence-base for a theory or practice (Begeny et al., 2021; Bernardo et al, 2018).

One example of a method to address at least some of the aforementioned issues is QuantCrit. QuantCrit offers a framework for critically examining the objectivity of quantitative research methods and algorithms that can skew data and increase interpretation errors that lead to more pseudoscience. Application of some basic tenets of QuantCrit – that numbers are not neutral, data cannot "speak for itself," statistical analyses have no inherent value, racism and other forms of systemic oppression are complex and not easily quantifiable, and the experiential knowledge of underrepresented groups should inform critical analyses (Garcia et al., 2017) – can help us engage critically with data or numbers that are presented to us as unquestionably "objective" or "true," but may in fact foster pseudoscience, academic neocolonialism, or racism.

Gaps and Future Research Directions

Further research is needed to ascertain the dangers of neuromyths. For example, Horvath et al. (2018) pointed out that scientific research has yet to demonstrate *how much* of an impact dispelling neuromyths would actually have on teacher practice or effectiveness. Similarly, in their systematic review of learning styles research, Newton and Salvi (2020) noted that past research has heavily relied on self-report rather than direct observation of educators in their classrooms. Directly measuring educators' actual behavior is critical to assessing the influence of neuromyths in education.

For example, perhaps some educators who report believing in learning styles theory are only demonstrating social desirability bias, and do not actually apply the theory in their classrooms. More research is also needed to examine effective interventions for dispelling neuromyths in academic instruction (Grospietsch & Lin, 2021), how long effects from such interventions last, or whether there is a risk of what some researchers are exploring as a *backfire effect* (i.e., the potential for opposing evidence to strengthen personal convictions; cf. Ferrero et al., 2016; Rousseau, 2021).

Recommendations

There is no simple solution to the problem of widespread adherence to unfounded beliefs, pseudoscience, and neuromyths. However, in addition to calling for more research, we wish to offer some general recommendations for educators and researchers that could lead to greater adoption of (a) practices that are likely to have large positive impacts on students and/or (b) methods to systematically evaluate instructional practice effectiveness.

1 Learning styles theory may be a special case of neuromyths that requires researchers' deeper engagement with the educational community because it may be confused with providing diverse instructional approaches that are individualized, differentiated, or multimodal (Macdonald et al., 2017). Thus, providing more clarification about the differences between learning styles theory and engaging students with individualized and/or multimodal instruction may be helpful.
2 We encourage cultivation of curiosity and cultural humility (see Tervalon & Murray-Garcia, 1998) – rather than negative judgment – regarding the reasons why people hold onto unfounded beliefs. Of course, dropping beliefs as soon as they are discovered to be false would prevent people from being wrong even a moment longer (see Harris, 2021). However, changing one's practices and beliefs can have serious negative effects on one's life and career, such as cognitive dissonance, feelings of having been "wrong" or harmful to past students, feeling previously misguided by respected colleagues or mentors, or weakened relationships with friends or coworkers (e.g., see The Clergy Project, 2023).
3 We encourage the use and understanding of rigorous research paradigms that extend beyond only using quantitative methods (e.g., qualitative and mixed-methods designs, as well as critical theory, can all support scientific understanding of effective instructional practices). Increased understanding of different paradigms, perspectives, and types of data, can help prevent the perpetuation of pseudoscience or the negative impacts of academic neocolonialism that come with the oversimplification and mischaracterization of quantitative findings.

Summary and Conclusion

Unfortunately, beliefs in neuromyths currently show no sign of decreasing anywhere in education or related to academic instruction. The key concern is not that a majority of educators have and will believe in neuromyths at some point; the concern is that high percentages of educators (and the general public; e.g., Fuertes-Prieto et al., 2020) continue to believe in neuromyths even after they have been debunked. Given existing research on how to minimize unfounded beliefs, one promising approach may be to provide some form of refutation, but it is still unclear which components of refutation are the most effective and socially valid, or how long their effects will last (Rousseau, 2021). Additionally, research in education and educational psychology continues to need more collaboration among researchers and practitioners (Begeny et al., 2018), and we argue that such collaboration is necessary to reduce instructional practices that are infeasible or pseudo-scientific. Though science cannot fix all of humanity's problems overnight, it – including critical and community-based collaborative science – holds great promise for enhancing educational effectiveness. As Carl Sagan (1980) said, "Science is not perfect. It's often misused. It is only a tool. But it is the best tool we have: Self-correcting, ever-changing, applicable to everything. With this tool, we vanquish the impossible" (p. 277).

References

Alatas, S. F. (2003). Academic dependency and the global division of labour in the social sciences. *Current Sociology*, *51*, 599–613.

Barberia, I., Tubau, E., Matute, H., & Rodríguez-Ferreiro, J. (2018). A short educational intervention diminishes causal illusions and specific paranormal beliefs in undergraduates. *PLoS One*, *13*, e0191907. 10.1371/journal.pone.0191907

Beals, K. P. (2022). Why we should not presume competence and reframe facilitated communication: a critique of Heyworth, Chan & Lawson. *Evidence-Based Communication Assessment and Intervention*, *16*, 66–76.

Begeny, J. C., Levy, R. A., Hida, R., Norwalk, K., Field, S., Suzuki, H., ... & Aguirre Burneo, C. (2018). Geographically representative scholarship and internationalization in school and educational psychology: A bibliometric analysis of eight journals from 2002-2016. *Journal of School Psychology*, *70*, 44–63.

Begeny, J. C., van Schalkwyk, G. J., Kim, E. K., Datu, J. A., Hida, R. M., Wang, J., & Grazioso, M. P. (2021). Engaging internationally to produce scholarship in school and educational psychology: A critical perspective. In R. G. Floyd & T. L. Eckert (Eds.), *Handbook of university and professional careers in school psychology* (pp. 212–228). Taylor & Francis.

Bernardo, A. B. I., Begeny, J. C., Earle, O. B., Ginns, D. S., Grazioso, M. P., Soriano-Ferrer, M., Suzuki, H., & Zapata, R. (2018). Internationalization within school and educational psychology: Perspectives about positive indicators, critical considerations, and needs. *Psychology in the Schools*, *55*, 982–992.

Blanchette Sarrasin, J., Riopel, M., & Masson, S. (2019). Neuromyths and their origin among teachers in Quebec. *Mind, Brain, and Education, 13*,100–109. 10.1111/mbe.12193

Busso D. S., & Pollack, C. (2015) No brain left behind: Consequences of neuroscience discourse for education. *Learning, Media and Technology, 40*, 168–186, DOI: 10.1080/17439884.2014.908908

Caroti, D., Adam-Troian, J., & Arciszewski, T. (2022). Reducing teachers' unfounded beliefs through critical-thinking education: A non-randomized controlled trial. *Applied Cognitive Psychology, 36*, 962–971.

Dekker, S., Lee, N. C., Howard-Jones, P., & Jolles, J. (2012). Neuromyths in education: Prevalence and predictors of misconceptions among teachers. *Frontiers in Psychology, 429*, 1–8. 10.3389/fpsyg.2012.00429

Deligiannidi, K., & Howard-Jones, P. A. (2015). The neuroscience literacy of teachers in Greece. *Procedia Social and Behavioral Science, 174*, 3909–3915. doi: 10.1016/j.sbspro.2015.01.1133

Eiser, J. R., Stafford, T., Henneberry, J., & Catney, P. (2009). "Trust me, I'm a scientist (not a developer)": Perceived expertise and motives as predictors of trust in assessment of risk from contaminated land. *Risk Analysis, 29*, 288–297. 10.1111/j.1539-6924.2008.01131.x

Ferrero, M., Garaizar, P., & Vadillo, M. A. (2016). Neuromyths in education: Prevalence among Spanish teachers and an exploration of cross-cultural variation. *Frontiers in Human Neuroscience, 10*, 496. 10.3389/fnhum.2016.00496

Fuentes, A., & Risso, A. (2015). Evaluación de conocimientos y actitudes sobre neuromitos en futuros/as maestros/as [Evaluation of knowledge and attitudes towards neuromyths in future teachers]. *Revista de Estudios e Investigación en Psicología y Educación, 6*, 193–198.

Fuertes-Prieto, M.Á., Andrés-Sánchez, S., Corrochano-Fernández, D., Urones-Jambrina, Carmen, Delgado-Martín, L., Herrero-Teijón, P., Ruiz, C. (2020). Pre-service teachers' false beliefs in superstitions and pseudosciences in relation to science and technology. *Science & Education, 29*, 1235–1254. 10.1007/s11191-020-00140-8

Furey, W. (2020). The stubborn myth of "learning styles" – State teacher-license prep materials peddle a debunked theory. *Education Next, 20*, 8–12.

Garcia, N. M., López, N., & Vélez, V. N. (2017). QuantCrit: Rectifying quantitative methods through critical race theory. *Race Ethnicity and Education, 21*, 149–157. 10.1080/13613324.2017.1377675

Gleichgerrcht, E., Luttges, B. L., Salvarezza, F., & Campos, A. L. (2015). Educational neuromyths among teachers in Latin America. *Mind, Brain, and Education. 9*, 170–178. doi: 10.1111/mbe.12086

Gonzalez, N. (2018). When evidence-based literacy programs fail. *Phi Delta Kappan, 100*, 54–58. 10.1177/0031721718815675

Grospietsch, F. & Mayer, J. (2018). Professionalizing pre-pervice biology teachers' misconceptions about learning and the brain through conceptual change. *Education Sciences, 8*, 1–23. 10.3390/educsci8030120

Grospietsch, F., & Mayer, J. (2019). Pre-service science teachers' neuroscience literacy: Neuromyths and a professional understanding of learning and memory. *Frontiers in Human Neuroscience, 13*, 20. 10.3389/fnhum.2019.00020

Grospietsch, F. & Mayer, J. (2020). Misconceptions about neuroscience – prevalence and persistence of neuromyths in education. *Neuroforum, 26,* 63–71. 10.1515/nf-2020-0006

Grospietsch, F. & Lins, I. (2021). Review on the prevalence and persistence of neuromyths in education—where we stand and what is still needed. *Frontiers in Education, 6,* 1–13. 10.3389/feduc.2021.665752

Harris, S. (2021, September 30). Belief and identity. In *Making Sense with Sam Harris.* Sam Harris. https://www.samharris.org/podcasts/making-sense-episodes/261-belief-identity

Hemsley, B., Bryant, L., Schlosser, R. W., Shane, H. C., Lang, R., Paul, D., Banajee, M., & Ireland, M. (2018). Systematic review of facilitated communication 2014–2018 finds no new evidence that messages delivered using facilitated communication are authored by the person with disability. *Autism & Developmental Language Impairments, 3,* 239694151882157.

Horvath, J. C., Donoghue, G. M., Horton, A. J., Lodge, J. M., & Hattie, J. A. C. (2018). On the irrelevance of neuromyths to teacher effectiveness: Comparing neuro-literacy levels amongst award-winning and non-award winning teachers. *Frontiers in Psychology, 9,* 1–5. 10.3389/fpsyg.2018.01666

Howard-Jones, P., Franey, L., Mashmoushi, R., & Liao, Y. (2009, September 2–5). *The neuroscience literacy of trainee teachers [Conference presentation].* British Educational Research Association Annual Conference, University of Manchester, England. https://www.bera.ac.uk/conference/bera-conference-2022

Kane, M. J., Core, T. J., & Hunt, R. R. (2010). Bias versus bias: Harnessing hindsight to reveal Paranormal belief change beyond demand characteristics. *Psychonomic Bulletin & Review, 17,* 206–212. 10.3758/PBR.17.2.206

Karakus, O., Howard-Jones, P. A., and Jay, T. (2015). Primary and secondary school teachers' knowledge and misconceptions about the brain in Turkey. *Procedia – Social and Behavioral Sciences, 174,* 1933–1940. doi: 10.1016/j.sbspro.2015.01.858

Kavale, K. A., & LeFever, G. B. (2007). Dunn and Dunn model of learning-style preferences: Critique of Lovelace meta-analysis. *The Journal of Educational Research, 101,* 94–97. https://www.jstor.org/stable/27548221

Lethaby, C., & Harries, P. (2016). Learning styles and teacher training: Are we perpetuating neuromyths?. *ELT Journal, 70,* 16–27. 10.1093/elt/ccv051

Macdonald, K., Germine, L., Anderson, A., Christodoulou, J., & McGrath, L. M. (2017). Dispelling the myth: Training in education or neuroscience decreases but does not eliminate Beliefs in neuromyths. *Frontiers in Psychology, 8,* 1–16.

Matute, H., Blanco, F., Yarritu, I., Diaz-Lago, M., Vadillo, M. A., & Barberia, I. (2015). Illusions of causality: How they bias our everyday thinking and how they could be reduced. *Frontiers in Psychology, 6,* 1–14.

Menz, C., Spinath, B., & Seifried, E. (2021). Where do pre-service teachers' educational psychological misconceptions come from?. *Zeitschrift für Pädagogische Psychologie, 35,* 143–156. 10.1024/1010-0652/a000299

Newton, P. M., & Miah, M. (2017). Evidence-based higher education – Is the learning styles 'Myth' important? *Frontiers in Psychology, 8,* 1–9. 10.3389/fpsyg.2017.00444

Newton, P. M., & Salvi, S. (2020). How common is belief in the learning styles neuromyth, and does it matter?. *Frontiers in Education, 5*, 1–14.

Organisation for Economic Co-operation and Development [OECD] (2007). *Understanding the brain: The birth of a learning science.* OECD Publications. https://www.oecd.org/education/ceri/38813448.pdf

Pasquinelli, E. (2012). Neuromyths: Why do they exist and persist?. *Mind, Brain, and Education, 6*, 89–96. 10.1111/j.1751-228X.2012.01141.x

Pei, X., Howard-Jones, P. A., Zhang, S., Liu, X., & Jin, Y. (2015). Teacher's understanding about the brain in East China. *Procedia – Social and Behavioral Sciences, 174*, 3681–3688. doi: 10.1016/j.sbspro.2015.01.1091

Rato, J., Abreu, A. M., & Castro-Caldas, A. (2013). Neuromyths in education: What is fact and what is fiction for Portuguese teachers?. *Educational Research, 55*, 441–453. doi: 10.1080/00131881.2013.844947

Richardson, M. (2018, August 20). An overview of evidence-based literacy interventions in North Carolina. *Education NC.* https://www.ednc.org/an-overview-of-evidence-based-literacy-interventions-in-north-carolina/

Rohrer, D., & Pashler, H. (2012). Learning styles: Where's the evidence?. *Medical Education, 46*, 634–635. 10.1111/j.1365-2923.2012.04273.x

Rousseau L. (2021). Interventions to dispel neuromyths in educational settings: A review. *Frontiers in Psychology, 12*, 1–12. 10.3389/fpsyg.2021.719692

Sagan, C. (1980). Who speaks for the earth? Cosmos. Season 1: Episode 13 https://www.organism.earth/library/document/cosmos-13)

Simmonds, A. (2014). *How neuroscience is affecting education: Report on teacher and parent Surveys.* London: Welcome Trust. https://wellcomecollection.org/works/txqphp6g\

Tervalon, M., & Murry-Garcia, J. (1998). Cultural humility versus cultural competence: A critical distinction in defining physician training outcomes in multicultural education. *Journal of Health Care for the Poor and Underserved, 9*, 117–125. 10.1353/hpu.2010.0233

Thalmayer, A. G., Toscanelli, C., & Arnett, J. J. (2021). The neglected 95% revisited: Is American psychology becoming less American?. *American Psychologist, 76*, 116–129.

The Clergy Project (2023). *Welcome to the clergy project.* https://clergyproject.org/

Torrijos-Muelas, M., González-Víllora, S., & Bodoque-Osma, A. (2021). The persistence of neuromyths in educational settings: A systematic review. *Frontiers in Psychology, 11*, 1–18.

van Dijk, W., & Lane, H. B. (2018). The brain and the US education system: Perpetuation of neuromyths. *Exceptionality, 28*, 16–29. 10.1080/09362835.2018.1480954

Vollmer, L. E., Gettinger, M., & Begeny, J. C. (2019). Preservice training in response to intervention (RTI): What are teacher education programs teaching?. *Journal of Applied School Psychology, 35*, 122–145.

Willingham, D. T., Hughes, E. M., & Dobolyi, D. G. (2015). The scientific status of learning styles theories. *Teaching of Psychology, 42*, 266–271. 10.1177/0098628315589505

10 Academic Interventions

Zachary C. LaBrot and Emily R. DeFouw

As many as 30% of youth experience reading, writing, or mathematics difficulties (U.S. Department of Education, 2011, 2020). Because of the educational disruptions due to the pandemic and national teacher shortage, these rates of academic difficulties are likely to increase, even if temporarily. In fact, the most recent Nation's Report Card conducted by the National Assessment of Educational Progress (NAEP) revealed substantial losses across both reading (3-point loss) and math (5-point loss) for US students compared to pre-pandemic years (NCES, 2022). Given these alarming rates of learning difficulties, it is imperative that educational professionals are prepared to deliver effective, evidenced-based academic interventions to ameliorate learning difficulties. While several academic interventions have been shown to improve reading, writing, and mathematics outcomes across various grade levels (e.g., Codding et al., 2011; Gillespie & Graham, 2014; Lee & Yoon, 2017), there also exist several questionable academic interventions.

These questionable practices generally have little to no empirical support but are widely disseminated and adopted by educational professionals. Given their widespread dissemination, education professionals often embrace and implement these practices to the detriment of the youth they serve. This is unsurprising, as questionable practices are often promoted in such a manner that they appear logical and even scientific as they play on natural human biases (Lilienfeld et al., 2012). As such, in this chapter, we'll explore three primary claims: 1) educational kinesiology enhances learning, 2) vision therapies improve academic outcomes, and 3) discovery learning is an effective academic remediation strategy.

Examining the Claims

Claim #1: Educational Kinesiology Enhances Learning

Educational kinesiology, also called perceptual-motor programs, is the practice of enhancing learning by having individuals engage in a series of

DOI: 10.4324/9781003266181-14

movements designed to integrate visual, auditory, and kinesthetic sensory input to promote learning, and therefore improve academic outcomes (Hyatt et al., 2009; Spaulding et al., 2010). The premise of educational kinesiology is that learning difficulties are caused by neurological processing deficits that interfere with perceptual and motor functioning and therefore impact academic learning. As such, the educational kinesiology approach involves training specific fine and gross motor movement exercises that purportedly integrate and improve neurological structures to improve learning. Various educational kinesiology treatment packages designed their approaches based on this premise to improve youths' academic outcomes (Hyatt et al., 2009). Brain Gym® International (BGI; Dennison & Dennison, 1994) is perhaps the most well-known educational kinesiology program that is extensively marketed and has garnered wide acceptance among educational professionals.

Educational kinesiology is based on the theories of neurological repatterning, mixed cerebral dominance, and perceptual-motor training (Hyatt, 2007). Neurological repatterning postulates that individuals must acquire certain motor skills during development to achieve appropriate neurological functioning and certain motor movements can properly shape underdeveloped neural pathways. Mixed cerebral dominance posits reading difficulties are attributable to the functioning of one hemisphere of the brain being predominant over the other. Various physical learning strategies (e.g., simultaneously saying the sounds of letters while tracing the letters) can purportedly integrate left- and right-brain functions. Finally, perceptual-motor training involves engaging in a variety of physical activities (e.g., walking on a balance beam) to improve perceptual-motor skills that inhibit learning (Hyatt, 2007; Spaulding et al., 2010). Although a comprehensive discussion of each of these is beyond the scope of this chapter, it is important to note that each of these theories has limited empirical support for their ability to specifically improve academic outcomes (Hyatt, 2007; Spaulding et al., 2010). However, the promise of improving learning quickly and simply, and its claimed foundations in neuroscience, make educational kinesiology an enticing approach to improving academic outcomes.

To date, limited current peer-reviewed studies have been published that evaluate the effectiveness of educational kinesiology programs on specific academic outcomes, while many have been published in non-referred journals. Although recent research is hard to find, several decades ago, Kavale and Mattson (1983) were able to conduct a meta-analysis of 180 studies evaluating the effects of educational kinesiology for improving reading and mathematics skills and overall academic achievement. Results indicated that educational kinesiology had no significant effects on mathematics, reading performance, or overall academic achievement.

More recently, Watson and Kelso (2014) evaluated the effects of the treatment used by Brain Gym® International for increasing academic engagement for three children with developmental disabilities in an after-school academic remediation clinic. Much like previous research, results of this study indicated that educational kinesiology was not effective for increasing academic engagement across the three participants. However, it is important to note that this study did not measure continued use of educational kinesiology techniques over time to determine their potential long-term effects.

Overall, the literature does not support the effectiveness of educational kinesiology for improving students' academic or related outcomes. Some peer-reviewed literature suggests that educational kinesiology may be beneficial for improving balance (Khalsa et al., 1988), response time (Sifft & Khalsa, 1991), and perceptual-motor skills (Cammisa, 1994). However, these outcomes are not indicative of reading, writing, or mathematics outcomes. Furthermore, these studies contained serious methodological flaws, such as limited description of procedures, poor treatment fidelity, and use of subjective outcome measures that fail to support the effectiveness of educational kinesiology (Hyatt, 2007; Spaulding et al., 2010). Although no published research has documented the direct harms of educational kinesiology, there are inherent issues with these approaches to ameliorating academic difficulties. Namely, the financial costs and time commitments associated with these approaches may interfere with a youth's ability to access otherwise effective academic assessment and intervention services.

Claim #2: Vision Therapies Improve Academic Outcomes

The primary premise of vision therapy, also called behavioral optometry, is that difficulties with visual processing and perception result in reading and writing difficulties. It is important to note that proponents of vision therapy are not suggesting that poor vision is the cause of reading difficulties (which can certainly be true); instead, the *processing* of written letters and words is problematic. As such, to address these issues, vision therapists recommend repeated practice in various eye movements and eye-hand coordination exercises to improve visual memory, visual discrimination, visual-spatial orientation, and visual-motor integration. These exercises purportedly improve visual-spatial processing, scanning, and locating; and they subsequently make one more receptive to reading and writing instruction (Handler & Fierson, 2011). The foundations of vision therapy are largely based on a series of clinical impressions as opposed to rigorous experimental studies (Barrett, 2009). Nevertheless, youth diagnosed with attention-deficit/hyperactivity disorder (ADHD), dyslexia, dyspraxia, and various behavioral difficulties are often referred for vision therapies to improve academic outcomes.

Tinted lenses, a form of vision therapy, have also been used to address a variety of reading difficulties associated with scotopic sensitivity syndrome (SSS), also known as Irlen Syndrome and Meares-Irlen Syndrome. SSS purportedly produces visual discomfort and subsequent reading difficulties due to light sensitivity and visual distortion. These visual difficulties can allegedly result in poor reading fluency, difficulty with reading comprehension, misreading words, skipping over words and entire lines of text, and reading avoidance (Handler & Fierson, 2011). Tinted lenses purportedly alleviate these visual difficulties by filtering uncomfortable light waves and therefore lead to improved reading outcomes. Much like educational kinesiology, the promise of an easy and relatively straightforward approach to addressing reading difficulties is enticing. Unsurprisingly, vision therapies are widely disseminated and touted as an effective approach for improving reading and related academic outcomes.

The effectiveness of vision therapies has been widely investigated. In a comprehensive review of the literature, Barrett (2009) ultimately concluded that there is no scientific evidence that various eye or eye-hand movement exercises result in improved academic outcomes for youth diagnosed with specific learning disorders (SLDs). Similarly, in a comprehensive technical report produced by the American Academy of Pediatrics, Handler and Fierson (2011) found vision therapies that incorporate visual-motor exercises do not result in improved reading outcomes for youth with and without SLDs. Handler and Fierson (2011) ultimately concluded that the existing literature base evaluating the effects of vision therapies does not support this approach as evidence-based for improving reading outcomes for youth with SLDs.

Much like vision therapies, tinted lenses also have limited to no convincing evidence to support their effectiveness for addressing academic difficulties. Hyatt et al. (2009) conducted a comprehensive review of three questionable educational practices, including tinted lenses. This review of 17 studies found that tinted lenses had little to no effects for improving letter identification, word recognition, reading fluency, or reading comprehension. Likewise, Handler and Fierson (2011) indicated studies evaluating the effectiveness of tinted lenses demonstrated no differences in reading accuracy, fluency, or comprehension for youth with reading difficulties (including those diagnosed with reading SLDs).

Although the comprehensive work of Hyatt et al. (2009) and Handler and Fierson (2011) highlight the ineffectiveness of vision therapies for improving academic outcomes, there have been some studies that support these approaches (e.g., Blaskey et al., 1990; O'Connor et al., 1990; Robinson & Conroy, 1990; Tran et al., 2004). However, these studies contained serious methodological flaws, such as a lack of control group, lack of control for the placebo effect, failure to determine group equivalence at pre- and post-test, experimenter bias, and irrelevant outcome measures (Handler & Fierson, 2011; Hyatt et al., 2009). Furthermore, several of these studies involved evaluating vision therapies while additional remedial supports (e.g., school-based academic interventions) were simultaneously occurring. In addition to these concerns, studies claiming the effectiveness of vision therapies are typically published in non-refereed journals. As such, it is difficult to determine whether the outcomes found in these studies were indeed attributable to the vision therapies, or various other extraneous variables. Moreover, the underlying theoretical foundations of vision therapies are themselves controversial (Handler & Fierson, 2011; Hyatt et al., 2009).

For example, although the primary tenet of vision therapies is that reading difficulties are attributable to visual processing issues, most studies do not conduct vision evaluations to verify these issues. As such, it is difficult (if not impossible) to verify that vision therapies can correct the underlying visual difficulties that purportedly lead to reading difficulties (Hyatt et al., 2009). Furthermore, SSS is not a recognized medical condition and cannot be detected by visual examinations (Handler & Fierson, 2011; Hyatt et al., 2009). So, it is unclear how this dubious diagnosis can be accurately assessed and linked to an effective intervention.

At this time, most research evaluating the effectiveness of vision therapies has focused on reading outcomes (Handler & Fierson, 2011; Hyatt et al., 2009). We were unable to identify any studies evaluating the effects of vision therapies on writing and mathematics outcomes. Given the relation between reading and other academic outcomes, it is unlikely that vision therapies lead to improved writing and mathematics outcomes. However, additional well-conducted research is needed to verify this assertion. Taken together, vision therapies to improve academic outcomes should be regarded with strong caution given their lack of research support and rigorous experimental studies. Much like educational kinesiology, the inherent problems with vision therapies are the cost and time needed for these procedures, which in turn may interfere with an individual's ability to seek effective academic services.

Claim #3: Discovery Learning Is an Effective Academic Remediation Strategy

Discovery learning is an academic teaching approach in which students are encouraged to uncover underlying principles and themes in academic tasks on their own. That is, students solve problems independently, as opposed to receiving direct instruction on how to solve the problems. This greater level of independence purportedly causes children to develop a deeper understanding of the topic they are studying, thus contributing to superior problem-solving skills (Alfieri et al., 2011; Klahr & Nigam, 2004). This concept is commensurate with that of Piaget's (1970) cognitive development theory in which youth act as "little scientists," taking active roles in their learning processes through exploration and experimentation.

The primary theoretical foundation of discovery learning is based on the cognitive constructivist model, in which learning is a process that occurs inside the mind. That is, the incorporation of novel information into a network of existing associations and knowledge will result in new connections (i.e., learning; Svinicki, 1998). This requires active learning, in which students are active participants compared to simply receiving instruction. It also involves meaningful learning, which posits that active learning leads to deeper connections which are more readily internalized and memorized by learners (Svinicki, 1998). Intuitively, these theories seem to make sense; as most individuals can recall times in which they learned something new from novel experiences without explicit teaching (e.g., young children quickly learn to avoid putting very hot food in their mouth after doing so). However, research in teaching and learning tends to suggest that discovery learning is less effective than direct instruction approaches (Klahr & Nigam, 2004; Lilienfeld et al., 2012; Mayer, 2004). Nevertheless, discovery learning has been utilized with many students in an attempt to improve mathematics and science outcomes (Klahr & Nigam, 2004), as well as remediate outcomes for struggling learners (Kroesbergen & Van Luit, 2003; Mahapatra, 2015). Discovery learning has been more widely applied as a teaching strategy than as a remediation strategy. Thus, we will first explore discovery learning as a teaching strategy.

First, it is important to understand the differences between pure discovery learning versus guided discovery learning, in which the former does not involve teacher prompting, questioning, and feedback while the latter does. To determine their relative effects, Klahr and Nigam (2004) experimentally compared pure discovery learning to direct instruction to improve students' science outcomes. Klahr and Nigam (2004) posited that discovery learning may have advantages to long-term, transferable learning. As such, this study compared two different stages of learning: (1) initial acquisition of the basic skill and (2) transfer and application of the basic skill. As Klahr and Nigam noted, research has failed to operationally define and experimentally evaluate discovery learning over the last 100 years (Winch, 1913). Given the lack of definition, they defined discovery learning as a "no teacher intervention" condition in that the teacher did not provide guiding questions or feedback. Children were tasked with selecting materials, exploring content, and conducting their own self-assessments. While children who received discovery learning demonstrated some gains, they were much smaller compared to students in the direct instruction condition. Klahr and Nigam (2004) concluded that direct instruction was "superior" to pure discovery learning in both skill acquisition and application. Similar results have continually been verified across the discovery learning literature base.

For instance, Mayer (2004) conducted a literature review examining the teaching of problem-solving rules, conservation strategies, and program concepts and found that pure discovery learning strategies quite simply did not improve learning outcomes. Likewise, Kirschner et al. (2006) also reviewed a series of well-controlled experimental studies evaluating the relative effects of pure discovery learning to direct instructional methods. Unsurprisingly, Kirschner et al (2006). found, across all reviewed studies, that guided instructional approaches were superior to unguided (i.e., pure discovery) for promoting students' learning outcomes. Finally, in a comprehensive meta-analysis, Alfieri et al. (2011) reviewed 108 studies comparing the effectiveness of pure discovery learning to direct instruction methods and found direct instruction methods were superior for promoting mathematics, science, problem solving, and verbal/social skills across children, adolescents, and adults. Although these studies offer overwhelming evidence that guided instructional approaches are superior to unguided, they do not necessarily suggest that discovery learning with guidance is an inferior teaching practice.

To address this specific line of inquiry, researchers have evaluated the relative effectiveness of guided discovery learning (also called assisted discovery learning) to more direct instructional approaches. Early experimental investigations clearly demonstrate that direct instructional methods are far more effective for improving students' science outcomes than guided discovery learning (Chen & Klahr, 1999; Kuhn & Dean, 2005; Strand-Cary & Klahr, 2008). Over time, other investigations tended to reveal similar findings. For example, in the second portion of their comprehensive meta-analysis, Alfieri et al. (2011) reviewed 56 research studies comparing guided discovery learning to more direct teaching approaches. Much like their findings evaluating pure discovery learning, Alfieri et al (2011). found that direct instructional methods were more effective than guided discovery learning in promoting outcomes in mathematics, computer skills, science, physical/motor skills, and social skills across children, adolescents, and adults.

Collectively, decades of research have clearly delineated that direct instruction is more effective than discovery learning (pure and guided) for promoting various academic outcomes, namely in the areas of mathematics and science. As such, it seems apparent that discovery learning is unlikely to have additional benefit for struggling learners. Nonetheless, some researchers have attempted to incorporate components of discovery learning into strategies designed to remediate academic difficulties, particularly in mathematics.

Kroesbergen and Van Luit (2003), for example, conducted a comprehensive meta-analysis of 58 mathematic intervention studies and examined the relative effectiveness of three intervention modalities: 1) direct instruction, 2) combined instructor- and self-instruction, and 3) discovery learning. Across these studies, the study demonstrated that students benefitted more from the first two modalities than the discovery learning modality when it came to promoting foundational mathematics skills, math facts, and problem-solving skills for students with and without SLDs, ADHD, emotional/behavioral difficulties, and developmental delays.

Given the preponderance of evidence, discovery learning strategies are unlikely to be helpful in the remediation of learning challenges (Alfieri et al., 2011; Kroesbergen & Van Luit, 2003; Mayer, 2004). Rather, direct instruction methods that include instructions, modeling, rehearsal, and feedback are needed to not only enhance teaching (Alfieri et al., 2011; Mayer, 2004) but also to remediate learning difficulties (Kroesbergen & Van Luit, 2003). This does not necessarily mean that discovery learning is completely ineffective. Instead, much of the reviewed research suggests that guided discovery learning (i.e., inclusion of teacher prompts, guidance, and feedback) can indeed be somewhat helpful for improving academic outcomes (Alfieri et al., 2011; Kirschner et al., 2006; Mayer, 2004). However, given the serious risk of students falling further behind, more direct instructional methods should be employed in the remediation of academic difficulties. To that end, discovery learning is likely more beneficial as an adjunctive approach as opposed to a singular teaching or intervention strategy (Honomichl & Chen, 2012; Klahr & Nigam, 2004; Lilienfeld et al., 2012).

Summary and Conclusion

Given the high rate of youths that experience learning difficulties, it is imperative that educational and psychological professionals are prepared to remediate these concerns and prevent the development of additional academic deficits. Numerous strategies have been developed and tested to address academic difficulties. However, some of these strategies (such as educational kinesiology, vision therapies, and discovery learning) have little to no empirical support for improving struggling learners' academic outcomes. Unfortunately, these strategies have been marketed and widely disseminated to parents, teachers, and other education professionals as simple and cost-effective solutions for academic difficulties. Therefore, it is critical that professionals be diligent, yet critical, consumers of peer-reviewed literature. Education and psychology professionals should also remain skeptical of new procedures designed to improve academic outcomes but keep an open mind to the possibility of their effectiveness. Furthermore, researchers should subject new procedures for improving academic outcomes to rigorous experimental evaluations to guide practice. Without these efforts, questionable and potentially harmful academic intervention practices may continue to thrive. For more about pseudoscience in learning see LaBrot and Dufrene (2019) in the book *Pseudoscience in Child and Adolescent Psychotherapy: A Skeptical Field Guide* (Hupp, 2019).

Fortunately, there exists a range of empirically supported practices for improving academic outcomes for struggling learners. School-based Response to Intervention (RtI) (Jimerson et al., 2016), for instance, involves early detection of at-risk learners and a continuum of effective interventions for remediating academic difficulties. RtI systems include three tiers of service that gradually intensify in assessment and intervention procedures at each tier (Fuchs & Fuchs, 2006). Consistent progress monitoring and targeted, evidence-based interventions are consistently implemented across all three tiers. Regardless the tier of intervention supports, instruction and intervention implementation should be delivered via direct instruction, with verbal and written instructions, modeling, rehearsal, and feedback. Furthermore, effective academic interventions should be conceptually rooted in assessment results and linked to students' learning level within the Instructional Hierarchy (Daly et al., 1996; Kupzyk & LaBrot, 2021; Kupzyk et al., 2023).

References

Alfieri, L., Brooks, P. J., Aldrich, N. J., & Tenenbaum, H. R. (2011). Does discovery-based instruction enhance learning?. *Journal of Educational Psychology, 103*(1), 1–18. 10.1037/a0021017

Barrett, B. T. (2009). A critical evaluation of the evidence supporting the practice of behavioural vision therapy. *Ophthalmic and Physiological Optics, 29*(1), 4–25. 10.1111/j.1475-1313.2008.00607.x

Blaskey, P., Scheiman, M., Parisi, M., Ciner, E. B., Gallaway, M., & Selznick, R. (1990). The effectiveness of Irlen filters for improving reading performance: A pilot study. *Journal of Learning Disabilities, 23*(10), 604–612. 10.1177/002221 949002301007

Cammisa, K. M. (1994). Educational kinesiology with learning disabled children: An efficacy study. *Perceptual and Motor Skills, 78*, 105–106. 10.2466/pms.1994. 78.1.105

Chen, Z., & Klahr, D. (1999). All other things being equal: Acquisition and transfer of the control of variables strategy. *Child Development, 70*(5), 1098–1120. 10.1111/1467-8624.00081

Codding, R. S., Burns, M. K., & Lukito, G. (2011). Meta-analysis of mathematic basic-fact fluency interventions: A component analysis. *Learning Disabilities Research & Practice, 26*(1), 36–47. 10.1111/j.1540-5826.2010.00323.x

Daly III, E. J., Lentz Jr., F. E., & Boyer, J. (1996). The instructional hierarchy: A conceptual model for understanding the effective components of reading interventions. School Psychology Quarterly, *11*(4), 369–386. 10.1037/h0088941

de los Santos, G., Hume, E. C., & Cortes, A. (2002). Improving the faculty's effectiveness in increasing the success of Hispanic students in higher education – pronto!. Journal of Hispanic Higher Education, *1*(3), 225–237. 10.1177/15381 92702001003003

Dennison, P. E., & Dennison, G. E. (1994). Brain Gym® teacher's edition – Revised. Ventura, CA: Edu-Kinesthetics.

Ducharme, J. M., & Shecter, C. (2011). Bridging the gap between clinical and classroom intervention: Keystone approaches for students with challenging behavior. School Psychology Review, *40*(2), 257–274. 10.1080/02796015. 2011.12087716

Fuchs, D., & Fuchs, L. S. (2006). Introduction to response to intervention: What, why, and how valid is it? Reading Research Quarterly, *41*, 93–99. https://www.jstor.org/stable/4151803

Gillespie, A., & Graham, S. (2014). A meta-analysis of writing interventions for students with learning disabilities. Exceptional Children, *80*(4), 454–473. 10.1177/0014402914527238

Handler, S. M., & Fierson, W. M. (2011). Joint technical report – learning disabilities, dyslexia, and vision. Pediatrics, *127*(3), e818–e856.

Honomichl, R. D., & Chen, Z. (2012). The role of guidance in children's discovery learning. Wiley Interdisciplinary Reviews: Cognitive Science, *3*(6), 615–622. 10.1002/wcs.1199

Hyatt, K. J. (2007). Brain Gym®: Building stronger brains or wishful thinking?. Remedial and Special Education, *28*(2), 117–124. 10.1177/0741932507028002 0201

Hyatt, K. J., Stephenson, J., & Carter, M. (2009). A review of three controversial educational practices: Perceptual motor programs, sensory integration, and tinted lenses. Education and Treatment of Children, *32*(2), 313–342. https://www.jstor.org/stable/42900024

Hupp, S. (2019). Pseudoscience in child and adolescent psychotherapy: A skeptical field guide. Cambridge University Press.

Jimerson, S. R., Burns, M. K., & VanDerHeyden, A. M. (2016). From response to intervention to multi-tiered systems of support: Advances in the science and practice of assessment and intervention. In S. R. Jimerson, M. K. Burns, & A. M. VanDerHeyden (eds.). Handbook of response to intervention. 2nd ed., pp. 1–6. New York: Springer.

Kavale, K. A., & Mattson, P. D. (1983). "One jumped off the balance beam": Meta-analysis of perceptual-motor training. Journal of Learning Disabilities, *16*, 165–173. 10.1177/002221948301600307

Khalsa, G. K., Morris, G. S. D., & Sifft, J. M. (1988). Effect of educational kinesiology on static balance of learning disabled students. Perceptual and Motor Skills, *67*, 51–54. 10.2466/pms.1988.67.1.51

Kirschner, P., Sweller, J., & Clark, R. E. (2006). Why unguided learning does not work: An analysis of the failure of discovery learning, problem-based learning, and experiential learning and inquiry-based instruction. Educational Psychologist, 41(2), 75–86.

Klahr, D., & Nigam, M. (2004). The equivalence of learning paths in early science instruction: Effects of direct instruction and discovery learning. Psychological Science, 15(10), 661–667. 10.1111/j.0956-7976.2004.00737.x

Kroesbergen, E. H., & Van Luit, J. E. (2003). Mathematics interventions for children with special needs: A meta-analysis. Remedial and Special Education, 24(2), 97–114. 10.1177/07419325030240020501

Kuhn, D., & Dean Jr., D. (2005). Is developing scientific thinking all about learning to control variables?. Psychological Science, 16(11), 866–870. 10.1111/j.1467-9280.2005.01628.x

Kupzyk, S., & LaBrot, Z. C. (2021). Teaching future school personnel to train parents to implement explicit instruction interventions. Behavior Analysis in Practice, 14(3), 856–872. 10.1007/s40617-021-00612-5

Kupzyk, S., LaBrot, Z. C., & Collins, M. (2023). An updated systematic review of parent tutoring literature. Education and Treatment of Children.

LaBrot, Z., & Dufrene, B. (2019). Learning. In S. Hupp (Ed), Pseudoscience in child and adolescent psychotherapy: A skeptical field guide (pp. 66–79). Cambridge University Press.

Lee, J., & Yoon, S. Y. (2017). The effects of repeated reading on reading fluency for students with reading disabilities: A meta-analysis. Journal of Learning Disabilities, 50(2), 213–224. 10.1177/0022219415605194

Lilienfeld, S. O., Ammirati, R., & David, M. (2012). Distinguishing science from pseudoscience in school psychology: Science and scientific thinking as safeguards against human error. Journal of School Psychology, 50(1), 7–36. 10.1016/j.jsp.2011.09.006

Mahapatra, S. (2015). Cognitive training and reading remediation. Journal of Education and Practice, 6(19), 57–63.

Mayer, R. E. (2004). Should there be a three-strike rule against pure discovery learning?. American Psychologist, 59, 14–19. 10.1037/0003-066X.59.1.14

National Center for Education Statistics [NCES] (2022). The Nation's report card: 2022 Mathematics & Reading Assessments. Institute of Education Sciences, U.S. Department of Education.

O'Connor, P. D., Sofo, F., Kendall, L., & Olsen, G. (1990). Reading disabilities and the effects of colored filters. Journal of Learning Disabilities, 23(10), 597–603. 10.1177/002221949002301006

Piaget, J. (1970). Piaget's theory. In P. Mussen (Ed.), Carmichael's manual of child psychology (Vol. 1, pp. 703–772). New York: John Wiley & Sons.

Robinson, G. L., & Conway, R. N. (1990). The effects of Irlen colored lenses on students' specific reading skills and their perception of ability: A 12-month validity study. Journal of Learning Disabilities, 23(10), 589–596. 10.1177/002221949002301005

Sifft, J. M., & Khalsa, G. C. K. (1991). Effect of educational kinesiology upon simple response times and choice response times. Perceptual and Motor Skills, 73, 1011–1015. 10.2466/pms.1991.73.3.1011

Spaulding, L. C., Mostert, M. P., & Beam, A. P. (2010). Is Brain Gym® an effective educational intervention?. Exceptionality, *18*, 18–30. 10.1080/093628309034 62508

Strand-Cary, M., & Klahr, D. (2008). Developing elementary science skills: Instructional effectiveness and path independence. Cognitive Development, *23*(4), 488–511. 10.1016/j.cogdev.2008.09.005

Svinkicki, M. D. (1998). A theoretical foundation for discovery learning. Advances in Physiology Education, *275*(6), 4–7. 10.1152/advances.1998.275.6.S4

Tran, K., Yu, C., Okumura, T., & Laukkanen, H. (2004). Effectiveness of an online computerized eye movement training program to improve oculomotor control in adult readers: A pilot study. Journal of Behavioral Optometry, *15*(5), 115–121.

U.S. Department of Education, Institute of Education Sciences, National Center for Education Statistics, National Assessment of Educational Progress (NAEP) (2020). Results from the 2019 Mathematics and Reading Assessments. Retrieved August 30, 2020 from https://www.nationsreportcard.gov/

U.S. Department of Education, Institute of Education Sciences, National Center for Education Statistics, National Assessment of Educational Progress (NAEP) (2011). Writing Assessment. Retrieved July 6, 2015 from https://nces.ed.gov/nationsreportcard/pdf/main2011/2012470.pdf

Watson, A., & Kelso, G. L. (2014). The effect of Brain Gym® on academic engagement for children with developmental disabilities. International Journal of Special Education, *29*(2), 75–83.

Winch, W. A. (1913). Inductive versus deductive methods of teaching. Baltimore: Warwick and York.

11   Working Memory Training

Sarah J. Conoyer, Kathrin E. Maki, and Jamie Haas

In everyday nomenclature, for many people, the concept of working memory (WM) is often associated with phone numbers because seven-plus-or-minus-two is often assumed to be the maximum amount of information that can be held by most people in this working metacognitive space. Yet, WM is a complex part of our memory system. WM is a key component of our cognitive architecture that functions as a mental workspace to manipulate information as part of learning, reasoning, and problem solving (Cowan, 2014). It has often been described as the notepad that allows individuals to store information being processed, requiring attentional resources to engage in such processing. There are different types of WM in that it can store and manipulate information that is verbal, numerical, visuospatial, or a combination of these information types (Chai et al., 2018; Klingberg et al., 2005), which have been found to be associated with different types of academic skills. For example, reading skills were shown to be related to verbal WM, and math computation and problem-solving tasks were shown to relate to visuospatial or numerical WM abilities (Cassidy et al., 2016). Students with academic difficulties or specific learning disabilities (SLDs) were more likely to exhibit a WM deficit than students with average academic skills (Horowitz et al., 2017). Thus, some have argued that WM training with students across a broad array of contexts has the potential to improve cognitive functioning and academic skills (e.g., Klingberg et al., 2002; Spencer-Smith & Klingberg, 2015).

Working memory (WM) training has often been recommended to increase memory or problem-solving skills. As technology has advanced, WM training has often been packaged as "brain training" in the form of games that can be accessed via the internet or mobile device. These types of games may include memorizing and recalling digits or words, recalling changing details in a story, or looking for patterns visually. Such training has become increasingly prevalent and accessible for both children and adults. These programs often claim that engaging in exercises or games will increase memory abilities that will assist with learning outcomes. As such,

DOI: 10.4324/9781003266181-15

some studies have suggested that cognitive functioning can be treated like a muscle that can be trained and improved (Colbert et al., 2018). Ultimately, proponents of WM training assert that an increase in students' WM ability will result in improvements in academic skills such as reading and math, given the documented relationships between WM and academic skills. This chapter will examine claims related to WM training programs. See also the "Brain Training and Intelligence" chapter (Schneider & Viskontas, 2023) in the book *Investigating Pop Psychology: Pseudoscience, Fringe Science, and Controversies* (Hupp & Wiseman, 2023).

Examining the Claims

Many WM training programs incorporate WM as a component of broader cognitive ability training programs, though we refer to them here as WM training programs for language consistency. These programs are readily available for everyday consumers with a quick internet search returning multiple online and face-to-face WM training programs for both children and adults. Many of the sites describe their curricula as brain-based training programs in which individuals engage in exercises to improve WM, memory broadly, attention, and general cognitive functioning, and they emphasize the positive outcomes associated with such training.

WM training programs typically report that their methods are widely used and research-based or "proven" to improve memory. Training programs often claim to improve WM, attention, and academic perform-ance for students, especially for students with attention-deficit/hyperactivity disorder (ADHD). Cogmed provides online WM training through exercises and games that are tailored with a Cogmed coach. Sessions may last from 20 to 50 minutes. The website purports that "anyone completing the training program with dedicated effort will see a significant effect on their working memory, attention, and cognitive performance" (Cogmed, 2022; section 5). The Cogmed website provides supportive quotes from various professionals including those with PhDs and MDs. It also reports over 200,000 users and indicates that the program is "scientifically proven" and effective in over 120 scientific articles. However, although various WM training company websites refer to research on their products, the research is often conducted by researchers affiliated with the company, suggesting a potential conflict of interest.

Evidence of Beliefs in Working Memory Training

There is considerable belief in the effectiveness of WM training programs. Such beliefs are evidenced by: (1) their widespread use, (2) theories about the causal nature of the associations between WM and academic skills, and (3) users' reporting of program effectiveness. Each of these points is discussed below.

WM training programs have effectively marketed their programs as evidenced by the fact that they are now a multi-billion-dollar industry with millions of consumers annually (Goghari et al., 2020). For example, one company reported over 100 million users (Lanius, 2022), and 33% of participants in a study of WM training programs reported using it at one point in their lives (Goghari et al., 2020). This overwhelming usage underscores the appeal of such programs to everyday consumers. To attract a large body of users, WM training programs use rhetoric and images focusing on young and healthy development (Lanius, 2022). The websites also include quotes from consumers and experts lending credence to the companies' claims and their programs' purported effectiveness.

WM training programs and other proponents of WM training emphasize that training WM can improve an individual's cognitive processing, and for children and adolescents, that processing is particularly important for academic performance. Several programs purport that cognitive training, and specifically WM training, will remediate the problem underlying academic difficulties, thereby leading to improvements in academic skills. Such claims may be based on research consistently demonstrating *relations* between specific cognitive abilities and academic skills. WM has been shown to be correlated with math computation (Villeneuve et al., 2019), reading fluency, and comprehension (Hajovsky et al., 2014). Supporters of WM training have asserted that the correlation between WM and academic skills suggests that WM deficits are *causing* academic difficulties. Furthermore, they have claimed remediating those deficits will therefore lead to improvements in academic skills (Klingberg et al., 2002; Spencer-Smith & Klingberg, 2015). Therefore, it may be intuitively appealing to attempt to remediate a potential underlying cognitive deficit to support students' academic skills.

Perceived effectiveness of WM training programs may also be due to participants' *beliefs* that the program is in fact effective. Many studies measuring the effectiveness of WM training have done so using self-report measures from individuals using these programs, with users reporting improvement in their memory (Goghari & Lawlor-Savage, 2018; Torous et al., 2016). Most individuals who used WM training programs perceived them as being "somewhat effective" and "somewhat supported" by research. Moreover, the longer participants used the WM training program, the more effective they reported it to be (Goghari et al., 2020). Relatedly, users' initial expectations of program effectiveness may influence perceptions of program effectiveness after completing the WM training (Boot et al., 2013; Shipstead et al., 2012). If users enter the program believing it will be effective and have invested significant resources (i.e., time and money), due to cognitive dissonance (Festinger, 1957), individuals may be more likely to rate the program as effective whether they notice an impact or not.

Critical Analysis of Working Memory Training Research

Critical evaluation of WM training claims and research is important given that significant student time and energy in and out of school, and parent and school financial resources are often devoted to these trainings. When examining the research from both sides of the WM training debate, it is important to understand the outcomes that are being evaluated. The main goal of WM training is to stimulate the "transfer" of abilities or skills from one domain like WM ability to another such as math skills (Titz & Karbach, 2014). Types of transfer can be defined as general training, and near and far transfer.

First, *general training* refers to training in one area of cognitive ability, in this case WM training, that results in an increase in overall cognitive ability, "*g*," or problem-solving skills. There is, however, disagreement regarding whether WM training is an effective general training approach to improve general cognitive ability. Often, cognitive ability assessments include WM tasks. Following WM training, individuals may exhibit gains in WM scores measured by these assessments without gains in "*g*" (overall cognitive functioning) or ultimately an increase in the student's capacity for problem solving in unfamiliar or academic tasks (Warne, 2020).

Second, *near transfer* is the demonstration of training effects on tasks that require a similar strategy that is taught through the training. That is, the individual is assessed on the same type of task on which they were trained. For example, if someone is trained to manipulate and recall a series of digits, then we would expect them to do well on the same digit recall task from training. This training often generalizes to other tasks on cognitive ability tests that require the student to recall digits.

Third, *far transfer* occurs when training on one task results in improvement or a change in a task that is unrelated to the training. An example of far transfer is training a student to complete a puzzle and then seeing improvement in their math word problem-solving skills. WM training seeks to affect far transfer such as increasing WM through training to ultimately positively impact academic problem solving in an area like math (Warne, 2020).

Evidence Used to Support Working Memory Training

Research has focused on the impact of WM deficits on academic skills and has shown that these deficits often impact specific clinical populations

(Wiest et al, 2022; Titz & Karbach, 2014). Moreover, as noted above, children with academic difficulties, particularly in math, consistently demonstrate WM deficits (Fuchs et al., 2020), highlighting the association between WM and academic skills. Students with grade-level or advanced academic skills were shown to perform better on WM tasks than students with academic difficulties (Titz & Karbach, 2014), and WM was shown to be related to academic skills, including later academic outcomes (Peng et al., 2018; Villeneuve et al., 2019).

WM training attempts to promote problem solving, planning, and attentional control (Melby-Lervåg et al., 2016) and has been shown to improve WM abilities in both children and adults (Melby-Lervåg & Hulme, 2013). WM training has resulted in immediate near-transfer effects on specific WM tasks and some long-term near-transfer effects such as increased fluid intelligence scores over a six-month period (Vernucci et al., 2022). Children who completed computerized WM training programs in school settings improved their WM abilities (Wiest et al., 2014, 2022). For example, Wiest et al. (2014) provided 34 students 20 hours of training embedded into a school day routine. They found that students made gains in WM and encoding, but pre-post effect sizes were larger for encoding skills compared to WM. However, the study did not include a control group to compare treatment effects. Yet, the authors suggested that WM training be incorporated into a Response to Intervention framework in schools to support students' WM abilities without directly assessing academic skills. They stated that the training "shows promise in remediating abilities that are significantly associated with academic performance" (p. 296). Spending 20 hours on a WM training program that *may be* associated with academic performance but has not been rigorously researched nor been shown to specifically improve academic skills when there are existing tools that target academic skills seems questionable, at the very least.

Despite proponents' assertions, there are several issues with these studies, including the questionable measurement of academic skills. Although some research has shown that WM training benefits were evident for those students with the most severe cognitive and academic weaknesses, the effects of these training programs have been shown to be dependent on the type of training used and individual characteristics of the sample (Titz & Karbach, 2014). Moreover, many of the studies demonstrating effects of WM training on academic skills did not include an active control group to compare WM training to traditional academic interventions; thus, it is unclear if WM training programs are effective compared to interventions directly targeting academic needs. Furthermore, some WM trainings have included academic skills training; thus, it is not clear if the academic skills training resulted in academic skills improvement or if WM training improved student academic skills.

Evidence against Working Memory Training

If WM deficits were the root cause of learning difficulties, including for students with ADHD or specific learning disability (SLD), then training that addresses these processes would consistently improve academic outcomes for students. However, research has not shown that to be the case. Although there is some support for the short-term near-transfer effects of WM training (Melby-Lervåg & Hulme, 2013), research supporting far-transfer and long-term outcomes is lacking. Most studies of WM training have not assessed academic skills (Wiest et al., 2014) or have found no far-transfer or long-term effects on reading or math measures (Vernucci et al., 2022).

By and large, WM training has not been shown to transfer to improvements in academic skills (Melby-Lervåg et al., 2013; Titz & Karbach, 2014). In a large meta-analysis, Melby-Lervåg et al. (2016) found that WM training, including commercially available WM training programs, did not result in improvements to academic skills compared to treatment control groups. That is, when students with WM deficits and academic difficulties received WM training, they may see improvements in WM; however, their academic skills (e.g., math computation) did not improve in concert. Such conclusions are not simply drawn from one or two studies; rather these conclusions were in response to multiple meta-analyses (e.g., Melby-Lervåg et al., 2013, 2016; Titz & Karbach, 2014), which provide strong evidence against WM training utility because they each combine the results of multiple studies.

Proponents of WM assessment and training have argued that it is necessary to understand the underlying cause of a student's academic difficulties to best support their needs (Peng & Swanson, 2022). However, this assertion is not supported by research given that students' academic skills have not consistently been shown to improve because of WM training. Given the lack of consistent support for the transfer of WM training to academic skills, some have also argued for combining WM training with academic skill intervention. Such interventions have been shown to improve academic skills (Fuchs et al., 2018; Kroesbergen et al., 2014), but generally not more than interventions targeting academic skills alone (Melby- Lervåg et al., 2016; Munez et al., 2022). Thus, combining WM training with academic skills intervention has not been shown to improve academic skills above and beyond traditional academic interventions.

Why People Believe Claims of Working Memory Training Effectiveness

Despite some evidence supporting short-term near transfer of WM training at best and contradicting evidence at worst, there are several reasons why people may believe claims supporting WM training including (1) the presentation of WM training programs as fun and effective games, (2) the goal of finding cures for significant difficulties/ disabilities, and (3) the desire for a causal explanation for learning difficulties.

Fun and Effective Games

WM training programs are often presented as games, puzzles, and other interesting activities. Such training programs are marketed as fun and engaging and are often implemented using technology (i.e., via computers or tablets), which is likely engaging for children given widespread use and interest in technology (Lanius, 2022). When compared to traditional academic interventions in schools that may include drill, practice, and repetition (which have all been shown to be effective intervention components; Ardoin et al., 2018; Zaslofsky et al., 2016), WM training is likely more appealing to both adults and children. In conjunction with framing WM training as games and fun activities, such programs use definitive language to make claims about the effectiveness of the program. Many websites claim their programs have been "proven" effective and provide research (some of which is methodologically faulty) only or primarily conducted by individuals with financial or other conflicts of interest in the research outcomes. Everyday consumers may not have the experience to critically consume and evaluate such research and therefore may consequently draw inappropriate conclusions regarding program effectiveness.

Curing Difficulties/Disabilities

Another reason individuals may believe claims of the effectiveness of WM training is because they may be inclined to seek alternative treatment for or want to cure significant difficulties or disabilities such as ADHD and SLD. Children with ADHD experience executive functioning difficulties, which often coincide with WM deficits. Although there are common treatment approaches for ADHD, such as behavioral techniques, these approaches are often inaccessible to many families (Manos et al., 2017). Some families are also uncomfortable with their child taking medication given the potential for adverse side effects (Cortese et al., 2013). As a result, some families may view WM training as a reasonable alternative approach. Further, as noted above, children with SLD commonly experience WM difficulties, and many believe it to be a hallmark of the disability (Berninger & Swanson, 2014). Thus, training and improving WM could be seen as a path to remediating the underlying problem that could ultimately cure the presenting symptoms (i.e., academic difficulties).

Causal Explanations

As part of efforts to remediate children's academic difficulties, parents and educators may seek causal explanations for why a child is exhibiting difficulties to (1) better understand the child's difficulties and (2) remediate the underlying problem. It's natural to seek explanations for why various phenomena occur, which likely takes the form of seeking causal explanations for children's academic difficulties. As noted above, WM ability has been shown to be associated with academic performance across a range of academic skills (Peng et al., 2018; Villeneuve et al., 2019). As such, when a child has trouble in math computation, for example, having information that the child also has low WM could help parents and educators feel that they better understand *why* the child is experiencing math difficulties. For some, the child's low WM ability is believed to cause math computation difficulties rather than other external factors. The logical next step from this perspective, then, is how this causal explanation can be used to inform academic intervention. Numerous evidence-based interventions for academic skills exist, particularly in reading and math (for example, see the National Center for Intensive Intervention); however, if a child has low WM that is associated with those academic difficulties, remediating the academic difficulties does not address the underlying problem.

As an analogy, if someone is experiencing weight loss due to Type 1 Diabetes, providing a highly caloric diet will not remediate the underlying hypo-insulin issues. Such an argument makes intuitive sense, but it is flawed. Remediating an underlying medical issue (e.g., hypo-insulin) transfers to remediating the symptoms associated with the condition. However, WM training has not been shown to transfer to improved academic skills (Melby-Lervåg et al., 2016).

Possible Harms of WM Training

Although there are likely few direct harms associated with WM training, the time, energy, and money spent on a questionable interventions can have negative consequences for students and other stakeholders. The school day is relatively short, with actual instructional time likely less than five hours per day (Dillon, 2019). Thus, it is critical that time spent in intervention to remediate students' academic difficulties is devoted to strategies and approaches that are evidence based (Cook & Cook, 2013).

That is, how much can students learn per unit of time? WM training programs are inherently inefficient given that they have not been shown to be effective for improving academic skills. Some have suggested that adding elements of WM training in conjunction with academic intervention may best support those with SLD and other academic difficulties (e.g., Fuchs et al., 2020). However, compared to direct academic intervention, such assertions have not been supported in classroom settings. WM training conducted in conjunction with academic interventions have been shown to be less effective than academic interventions alone (Munez et al., 2022).

Multiple WM training programs require a subscription and have turned into a multi-billion-dollar industry. Schools have finite financial resources, particularly in communities in lower socioeconomic neighborhoods (Yang & Lee, 2022). There is also the non-financial cost of students' academic skills not improving due to not receiving effective intervention, which has significant implications for those individual students. Students with academic difficulties are less likely to graduate from high school, attend college, and are more likely to earn less in adulthood (U.S. Bureau of Labor Statistics, 2019). Could observed shortcomings of WM training be due to measurement issues, inadequate dosage, or other strategy shortcomings that could be improved upon with continued research? The very nature of science involves the evolving examination of phenomena in response to research evidence. Currently, the evidence does not support WM training for improving academic skills. Thus, educators should advocate for implementation of research-supported academic interventions given the significant academic needs and limited resources to meet those needs.

Summary and Conclusion

WM training purports to address the underlying cause of children's academic difficulties rather than simply the symptom (i.e., the academic difficulty itself). Such framing intuitively appeals to researchers, educators, and families in search of solutions to improve children's and youth's academic skills. However, although there is evidence supporting the near transfer of WM, research has not supported the utility of WM for improving cognitive ability or academic skills (i,e., far transfer). Yet, there are numerous evidence-based interventions directly targeting academic skills (see the Postscript of this book). School psychologists must continually advocate for implementation of evidence-based practices to support approaches that are most likely to confer benefit to students. In the case of WM training, educators should focus efforts on directly intervening with academic skills rather than attempting to train WM, particularly given the need for intervention efficiency due to limited resources.

References

Ardoin, S. P., Binder, K. S., Zawoyski, A. M., & Foster, T. E. (2018). Examining the maintenance and generalization effects of repeated practice: A comparison of three interventions. Journal of School Psychology, *68*, 1–18. 10.1016/j.jsp. 2017.12.002

Berninger, V. W., & Swanson, H. L. (2014). Diagnosing and treating specific learning disabilities in reference to the brain's WM system. In H. L. Swanson, K. R. Harris, & S. Graham (Eds.), Handbook of learning disabilities (pp. 307–325). The Guilford Press.

Boot, W. R., Simons, D. J., Stothart, C., and Stutts, C. (2013). The pervasive problem with placebos in psychology: Why active control groups are not sufficient to rule out placebo effects. Perspectives on Psychological Science, *8*, 445–454. 10.1177/1745691613491271

Cassidy, S., Roche, B., Colbert, D., Stewart, I., & Grey, I. M. (2016). A relational frame skills training intervention to increase general intelligence and scholastic aptitude. Learning and Individual Differences, *47*, 222–235. 10.1016/j.lindif. 2016.03.001

Chai, W. J., Abd Hamid, A. I., & Abdullah, J. M. (2018). Working memory from the psychological and neurosciences perspectives: A review. Frontiers in Psychology, *9*. Article 401. 10.3389/fpsyg.2018.00401

Cogmed (2022). Cogmed. https://www.cogmed.com/

Colbert, D., Tyndall, I., Roche, B., & Cassidy, S. (2018). Can SMART training really increase intelligence? A replication study. Journal of Behavioral Education, *27*, 509–531. 10.1007/s10864-018-9302-2

Cook, B. G. & Cook. S. C. (2013). Unraveling evidence-based practices in special education. The Journal of Special Education, *47*(2), 71–82. 10.1177/00224 66911420877

Cortese, S., Holtmann, M., Banaschewski, T., Buitelaar, J., Coghill, D., Danckaerts, M., Dittmann, R. W., Graham, J., Taylor, E., & Sergeant, J. (2013). Practitioner review: Current best practice in the management of adverse events during treatment with ADHD medications in children and adolescents. The Journal of Child Psychology and Psychiatry, *54*, 227–246. 10.1111/jcpp.12036

Cowan, N. (2014). Working memory underpins cognitive development, learning, and education. Educational psychology review, *26*(2), 197–223. 10.1007/s10648-013-9246-y

Dillon, J. J. (2019). Inside today's elementary schools: A psychologist's perspective. Springer.

Festinger, L. (1957). A theory of cognitive dissonance.Evanston, IL: Row, Peterson.

Fuchs, L., Fuchs, D., Seethaler, P. M., Barnes, M. A. (2020). Addressing the role of working memory in mathematical word-problem solving when designing intervention for struggling learners. ZDM Mathematics Education 52, 87–96. 10.1007/s11858-019-01070-8

Fuchs, D., Hendricks, E., Walsh, M. E., Fuchs, L. S., Gilbert, J. K., Tracy, W. Z., … Peng, P. (2018). Evaluating a multidimensional reading comprehension program and reconsidering the lowly reputation of tests of near-transfer. Learning Disabilities Research & Practice, *33*(1), 11–23. 10.1111/ldrp.12162

Goghari, V. M., Krzyzanowski, D., Yoon, S., Dai, Y., & Toews, D. (2020). Attitudes and beliefs toward computerized cognitive training in the general population. Frontiers in Psychology, *11*, Article 503. 10.3389/fpsyg.2020.00503

Goghari, V. M., & Lawlor-Savage, L. (2018). Self-perceived benefits of cognitive training in healthy older adults. Frontiers in Aging Neuroscience, *10*. Article 112. 10.3389/fnagi.2018.00112

Hajovsky, D. B., Reynolds, M. R., Floyd, R. G., Turek, J. J., & Keith, T. Z. (2014). A multigroup investigation of latent cognitive abilities and reading achievement relations. School Psychology Review, *43*(4), 385–406. 10.1080/02796015.2014.12087412

Hardy, J. L., Nelson, R. A., Thomason, M. E., Sternberg, D. A., Katovich, K., Farzin, A., & Scanlon, M. (2015). Enhancing cognitive abilities with comprehensive training: A large, online randomized, active-controlled trial. PLoS ONE, *10*(9), e0134467. 10.1371/journal.pone.0134467

Horowitz, S. H., Rawe, J., & Whittaker, M. C. (2017). The state of learning disabilities: Understanding the 1 in 5. New York: National Center for Learning Disabilities. https://www.ncld.org/research/state-of-learning-disabilities

Hupp, S., & Wiseman, R. (2023). Investigating pop psychology: Pseudoscience, fringe science, and controversies. Routledge.

Klingberg, T., Fernell, E., Olesen, P. J., Johnson, M., Gustafsson, P., Dahlström, K., ... & Westerberg, H. (2005). Computerized training of working memory in children with ADHD-a randomized, controlled trial. Journal of the American Academy of Child & Adolescent Psychiatry, *44*(2), 177–186. 10.1097/00004583-200502000-00010

Klingberg, T., Forssberg, H., & Westerberg, H. (2002). Training of working memory in children with ADHD. Journal of Clinical and Experimental Neuropsychology, *24*, 781–791. 10.1076/jcen.24.6.781.8395.

Kroesbergen, E. H., van't Noordende, J. E., & Kolkman, M. E. (2014). Training WM in kindergarten children: Effects on WM and early numeracy. Child Neuropsychology, *20*(1), 23–37. 10.1080/09297049.2012.736483.

Lanius, C. (2022) Rhetoric of social statistics: Statistical persuasion and argumentation in the Lumosity memory wars. Rhetoric Review, *41*(1), 59–72. 10.1080/07350198.2021.2002070

Maki, K. E. & Hammerschmidt-Snidarich, S. (2022). Reading fluency intervention dosage: A novel research synthesis. Journal of School Psychology, *92*, 148–165. 10.1016/j.jsp.2022.03.008

Manos, M. J., Giuliano, K., & Geyer, R. (2017). ADHD: Overdiagnosed and overtreated, or misdiagnosed and mistreated?. Cleveland Clinic Journal of Medicine, *84*, 873–880. 10.3949/ccjm.84a.15051

Melby-Lervåg, M., & Hulme, C. (2013). Is WM training effective? A meta-analytic review. Developmental Psychology, *49*, 270–291. 10.1037/a0028228

Melby-Lervåg, M., & Hulme, C. (2016). There is no convincing evidence that WM training is effective: A reply to Au et al. (2014) and Karbach and Verhaeghen

(2014). Psychological Bulletin Review, *23*, 324–330. 10.3758/s13423-015-0862-z

Melby-Lervåg, M., Redick, T. S., and Hulme, C. (2016). WM training does not improve performance on measures of intelligence or other measures of "far transfer": Evidence from a meta-analytic review. Perspectives in. Psychological Science, *11*, 512–534. 10.1177/1745691616635612

Munez, D., Lee, K., Bull, R., Khng, K. H., Cheam, F., & Rahim, R. A., (2022). Working memory and numeracy training for children with math learning difficulties: Evidence from a large-scale implementation in the classroom. Journal of Educational Psychology, *114*(8), 1866–1880. 10.1037/edu0000732

Peng, P., Barnes, M., Wang, C., Wang, W., Li, S., Swanson, H. L., Dardick, W., & Tao, S., (2018). A meta-analysis on the relation between reading and WM. Psychological Bulletin, *144*, 48–76. 10.1037/bul0000124

Peng, P. & Swanson, H. L. (2022). The domain-specific approach of WM training. Developmental Review, *65*. 10.1016/j.dr.2022.101035

Schneider, M. J., & Viskontas, I. V. (2023). Brain training and intelligence. In S. Hupp and R. Wiseman (Eds), Investigating pop psychology: Pseudoscience, fringe science, and controversies (pp. 66–74). Routledge.

Shipstead, Z., Redick, T. S., & Engle, R. W. (2012). Is WM training effective?. Psychological Bulletin, *138*, 628–654. 10.1037/a0027473

Spencer-Smith, M., & Klingberg, T. (2015). Benefits of a working memory training program for inattention in daily life: A systematic review and meta-analysis. PLoS ONE, *10*(3), e0119522. 10.1371/journal.pone.0119522

Titz, C., & Karbach, J. (2014). Working memory and executive functions: Effects of training on academic achievement. Psychological Research, *78*(6), 852–868. https://doi.org/10.1007/s00426-013-0537-1

Torous, J., Staples, P., Fenstermacher, E., Dean, J., & Keshavan, M. (2016). Barriers, benefits, and beliefs of brain training smartphone apps: An internet survey of younger US consumers. Frontiers of Human Neuroscience, *10*. Article 180. 10.3389/fnhum.2016.00180

U.S. Bureau of Labor Statistics (2019). Retrieved from: http://www.bls.gov/news.release/hsgec.t01.htm

Vernucci, S., Canet-Juric, L., & Richard's, M. M. (2022). Effects of working memory training on cognitive and academic abilities in typically developing school-age children. Psychological Research. 10.1007/s00426-022-01647-1

Villeneuve, E. F., Hajovsky, D. B., Mason, B. A., & Lewno, B. M. (2019). Cognitive ability and math computation developmental relations with math problem-solving: An integrated, multi-group approach. School Psychology, *34*(1), 96–108. https://psycnet.apa.org/doi/10.1037/spq0000267

Warne, R. T. (2020). In the know: Debunking 35 myths about human intelligence. Cambridge University Press.

Wiest, G. M., Rosales, K. P., Looney, L., Wong, E. H., & Wiest, D. J. (2022). Utilizing cognitive training to improve working memory, attention, and impulsivity in school-aged children with ADHD and SLD. Brain Sciences, *12*(2), Article 141. 10.3390/brainsci12020141

Wiest, D. J., Wong, E. H., Minero, L. P., & Pumaccahua, T. T. (2014). Utilizing computerized cognitive training to improve working memory and encoding: Piloting a school-based intervention. Education, *135*(2), 264–27

Yang, M., & Lee, H. J. (2022). Do school resources reduce socioeconomic achievement gap? Evidence from PISA 2015. International Journal of Educational Development, *88.* 10.1016/j.ijedudev.2021.102528

Zaslofsky, A. F., Scholin, S. E., Burns, M. K., & Varma, S. (2016). Comparison of opportunities to respond and generation effect as potential causal mechanisms for incremental rehearsal with multiplication combinations. Journal of School Psychology, *55,* 71–78. 10.1016/j.jsp.2016.01.001

Part V

Working with Specific Populations and Problems

12 Neurodevelopmental Disorders

Angela Capuano and Kim Killu

Neurodevelopmental disorders are a category of disorders first present in childhood that affect development, such as autism spectrum disorder (ASD), intellectual disability, attention-deficit/hyperactivity disorder (ADHD), communication disorders, and learning disorders. Caregivers often feel overwhelmed when considering the range of available treatments, as there are many possible options (Schreck, 2014). Demand for treatments has increased, including both evidence-based and pseudoscientific practices (Metz et al., 2015), and pseudoscientific practices remain popular despite ample evidence of their ineffectiveness (Jacobson et al., 2015). Of the many dubious practices, those chosen for this chapter are popular (Green et al., 2006), likely to be encountered in school settings, and currently available to consumers.

For example, proponents of sensory integration claim to alter sensory deficits by engaging children in motor learning and purposeful activity (Schoen et al., 2022). Similarly, proponents of auditory integration claim that challenges arise from a condition known as hyperacusis, or sensitivity to sounds, and that training remediates these difficulties by exercising the inner muscles of the ear through specially attenuated sounds (Berkell et al., 1996). Proponents of another dubious practice, facilitated communication (FC), claim that manual assistance from a specially trained assistant helps children communicate (Jacobson et al., 1995). This chapter will examine claims related to all three of these approaches.

Examining the Claims

Sensory Integration

Sensory integration is a form of therapy used to treat presumed sensory dysfunctions. The therapy, developed by A. Jean Ayres, "is intended to focus directly on the neurological processing of sensory information as a foundation for learning of higher-level (motor or academic) skills" (Baranek, 2002, p. 406). Different sensory systems (e.g., vestibular, audio,

DOI: 10.4324/9781003266181-17

and visual) develop together, and, as such, therapy attempts to integrate these systems through motor learning and purposeful activity in order to remediate centralized deficits in sensory processing (Roley et al., 2007). Activities done in therapy are said to emerge dynamically between the therapist and child in a play-based manner (Schoen et al., 2022) and include approaches such as swinging, crawling through tunnels, bouncing on a ball, joint compressions, and brushing skin with a surgical brush. By engaging in these activities, children's nervous systems are enhanced to be better able to organize and use sensory input from the environment. Sensory integration interventions come in different variations with the most well-known being Ayres' Sensory Integration (ASI), termed sensory integration therapy (SIT) (Schoen et al., 2022). SIT is popular, with 50% of pediatric occupational therapists reporting using some sensory-based interventions (Williames & Erdie-Lalena, 2009). As sensory difficulties are purported to be very prevalent in neurodevelopmental disorders, their amelioration is one of the most-requested targets of treatment and often used by therapists working with students with ASD in public schools (Schaaf, 2011).

Case studies of sensory integration show some promise in improving sensory processing (Schaaf et al., 2012) and scores on parent-rated goal attainment scales (Clark et al., 2019; Parham et al., 2019). Group studies have shown improvement in ratings of sensory problems in children with ASD (Fazlioğlu & Baran, 2008) and ratings of motor coordination, nonverbal cognitive abilities, and sensory-motor abilities (Iwanaga et al., 2014). Single case studies show improvement in some motor skills (Andelin et al., 2021) and improvements in behavior regulation (Roberts et al., 2007). However, these improvements might be complicated by the concurrent removal of aversive stimuli, which may be responsible for reductions in the unwanted behavior. In recent years, there has been an increase in randomized controlled trials of SIT showing some improvement in social responsiveness (Pfeiffer et al., 2011), reduction of sensory problems (Kashefimehr et al., 2018; Pfeiffer et al., 2011), and achievement of parent-selected goals (Omairi et al., 2022; Schaaf et al., 2013).

Despite some promising results, research on SIT has been criticized for lacking methodological rigor (Addison et al., 2012; Schaaf, 2011), not being of high scientific quality (Schaaf et al., 2018), and failing to provide clear descriptions of the activities used (Mills et al., 2020). There are several additional critiques of the SIT research worth noting. First, several conceptual questions remain unanswered. For example, there is no conclusive evidence that children with sensory-based problems have a disorder associated with the brain's sensory pathways (e.g., sensory processing disorder), and there exists no universally accepted framework for a disorder and how such a disorder might be associated with ASD and other neurodevelopmental disorders (see Zimmer et al., 2012). Second, serious methodological concerns exist that limit study conclusions and generalizability of findings (Baranek, 2002). For example, the overreliance on parent-report measures to assess outcomes is problematic. Using outcome measures involving subjective parent reports might lead to positive ratings through expectancy effects (Ashburner et al., 2014; Baranek, 2002). Third, the literature lacks consistency on how to define sensory integration and SIT. Furthermore, there have been few descriptions of the exact activities associated with SIT (Addison et al., 2012; Schaaf, 2011). Although there have been efforts recently to standardize ASI (Parham et al., 2011; Schaaf & Blanche, 2011; Schaaf et al., 2012), research has failed to use manualized approaches that aid in intervention fidelity or assess fidelity altogether (Roley et al., 2007; Schaaf et al., 2018). Finally, high-quality studies consistently indicate SIT to be ineffective at reducing challenging behaviors associated with ASD (Davis et al., 2011; Watkins & Sparling, 2014), especially when compared to behaviorally based treatments (Addison et al., 2012; Lydon et al., 2017).

Although some researchers and many practitioners believe that SIT is evidence-based (Schoen et al., 2022), others disagree (Camarata et al., 2020; Smith et al., 2016; Stevenson, 2019; Williames & Erdie-Lalena, 2009). The American Academy of Pediatrics has stated that sensory-based therapies used with children with developmental disorders lack evidence (Zimmer et al., 2012). More recently, The National Standards Project of the National Autism Center categorized sensory-based interventions as *Unestablished*, meaning there is little or no evidence of their effectiveness (National Autism Center, 2015).

Auditory Integration

Auditory Integration Training (AIT) was developed by French oto-laryngologist Guy Berard in the 1960s and was popularized by a mother's 1991 memoir claiming that AIT led to her child miraculously recovering from ASD (Edelson et al., 1999; Mudford & Cullen, 2016). Following the publication of the memoir, AIT gained widespread popularity in the United States (Link, 1997; Mudford & Cullen, 2016) and was used to treat problems associated with ASD. AIT assumes a child's learning problems (e.g., academic, behavioral, and social skills deficits) are a function of oversensitive or hypersensitive hearing. Proponents of AIT claim that the brain is retrained when the individual listens to attenuated sounds, exercising ear muscles leading to less sensitivity to certain frequencies (LaFrance et al., 2015; Link, 1997). AIT consists of two 30-minute sessions over a total of 10 hours (Dawson & Watling, 2000; Mudford & Cullen, 2016), spaced out over a 10- to 20-day period

(Edelson et al., 1999). AIT has been used to address many aspects of ASD, such as development of speech, reduced hyperactive and impulsive behaviors, enhanced behavioral flexibility, and improved eye contact, social communication, listening, and attention (Brown, 1999). However, many view this theory as being outside realistic parameters of the human auditory system (Gravel, 1994; Tharpe, 1999).

There is a dearth of research on AIT (Parr, 2010), particularly involving randomized controlled trials (Mudford & Cullen, 2016). Most research on AIT was conducted in the 1990s and is in the form of case studies with small samples of participants. Investigators of these AIT case studies claim to show rapid and significant changes in children's functioning (Brown, 1999). In experiments that included control groups or placebo conditions, there was improvement noted on self-report measures of auditory and behavioral functioning (Edelson et al., 1999; Rimland & Edelson, 1995). A more recent study suggests children with ASD benefit from AIT by improved autonomic outcomes and reduced sound sensitivity (Sokhadze et al., 2016). Other studies suggest that AIT has long-term beneficial effects such as improved IQ scores, improved behaviors, and reductions in the severity of ASD symptoms (Bettison, 1996). Recent studies of AIT have examined improvement in biological factors that may or may not be related to ASD (Al-Ayadhi et al., 2018, 2019).

Despite the early promising results of some AIT research, many studies have failed to replicate similar findings. Some studies have found no significant differences in ASD symptoms after AIT (Gillberg et al., 1997; Link, 1997) or noted slightly worse functioning following AIT (Link, 1997). Other research established the control treatment to be superior to AIT (Mudford et al., 2000). LaFrance et al. (2015) found AIT to be ineffective in the treatment of motor and vocal stereotypy of a young child with ASD. Moreover, literature reviews have found that both AIT groups and control groups show improvement, suggesting that AIT alone may not be responsible for participants' improvement, and that studies indicating positive effects are often methodologically flawed (Dawson & Watling, 2000). Finally, systematic reviews reveal mixed results (Rossignol, 2009; Sinha et al., 2011).

Professional organizations and scholars have criticized the methods, analyses, and results of studies finding positive effects of AIT (e.g., using statistical procedures overly favorable to finding significant results) (American Speech-Language Hearing Association, 2004; Gillberg et al., 1998; Goldstein, 2003; Howlin, 1997; Sinha et al., 2011; Tharpe, 1999). In addition, some AIT studies have not properly matched the experimental and control groups, and, thus, the AIT groups had more room to improve on outcome measures; or the benefits of AIT may be due to the placebo effect as the caregivers in the studies expected there to be a positive effect of AIT (Siegel & Zimnitzky, 1998; Sokhadze et al., 2016). Finally, most

AIT studies have been in the form of case studies or anecdotal reports (Tharpe, 1999), which are subjective and biased, inconsistent, and lack conclusive evidence about the effectiveness of treatment (Green, 1996).

AIT remains unsupported (Dawson & Watling, 2000; Goldstein, 2000, 2003; Link, 1997; Mudford & Cullen, 2016; Parr, 2010), and possibly harmful to children's hearing (Berkell et al., 1996; Gravel, 1994; Mudford et al., 2000). Various professional organizations have argued against the use of AIT, such as the American Speech-Language Hearing Association (2004) and the American Academy of Pediatrics (1998). The National Standards Project, of the National Autism Center, lists AIT as an *Unestablished* intervention, which indicates that AIT produces no change in the symptoms or severity of ASD (NAC, 2015).

Facilitated Communication

FC (also referred to as "assisted typing," supported typing," and "spelling to communicate") involves a collection of methods that serve to provide manual assistance to a nonverbal individual to communicate with others. These methods involve an adult facilitator who uses manual prompting (e.g., holding or supporting the hand, wrist, or forearm of an individual) as the individual appears to spell out messages. With another similar method, the Rapid Prompting Method (RPM), a facilitator holds a letter board and provides a quick succession of verbal prompts to elicit communicative responses. In practice, RPM resembles the process used in FC. In any of these methods, the facilitator (i.e., the adult providing the manual support) is not supposed to influence what is typed, but rather, serves as the mechanism to augment the communication of the individual (e.g., by steadying the hand, providing the prompts, holding the letter board. The content typed out is assumed to be the thoughts of the individual receiving assistance and the individual's language and communication skills are supposedly revealed through the process.

FC emerged in Australia in the early 1970s when Rosemary Crossley used FC with several children with communication issues and physical disabilities (Crossley & McDonald, 1980). Douglas Biklen introduced FC in the United States in the 1990s as an intervention for individuals with ASD and intellectual disabilities (Biklen, 1990). Biklen maintained that individuals with ASD are affected by dyspraxia, a neurological disorder that affects speech production. FC, it was claimed, allows these individuals to overcome their communication challenges (Biklen, 1990; Biklen et al., 1992). The communication content (e.g., concepts, vocabulary) generated through Biklen's initial investigations was reportedly advanced, in stark contrast to the social, cognitive, and communicative challenges typically faced by individuals with ASD (Green & Shane, 1994). The use of FC expanded beyond those with ASD to intellectual and other developmental disabilities (Biklen & Schubert, 1991).

To date, the evidence presented by advocates of FC has been largely anecdotal or testimonial with very little attention paid to scientific integrity. Much of the FC research can be described as descriptive, rather than experimental. As an example, an investigation by Biklen et al. (1995) to determine authorship of text was designed to generate rather than test hypotheses. Publications promoting FC are largely outside of the peer-reviewed literature and often found in mainstream media outlets and the Internet. These representations of FC have been described as selective, incomplete, and inaccurate (Jacobson et al., 1995). Biklen (1993) argued that using scientific methods to study the efficacy of FC was unethical. He and others have also criticized experimental investigations of FC (Duchan, 1993) noting the nature of these investigations results in anxiety or an erosion of the relationship between the individual and facilitator thus impacting performance. He further argued that the facilitators in these experimental studies had not been properly trained and the individuals with disabilities did not have sufficient experience with FC.

Upon Biklen's introduction of FC in the United States, its use spread quickly. He established the Facilitated Communication Institute at Syracuse University, still in operation today (although now renamed the Institute on Communication and Inclusion), which quickly became the hub for training scores of therapists. Some parents were overjoyed when presented with the typed communications from their child, with often meaningful, loving words; words they had never heard before from their child. Some parents were convinced that their children were gifted and even psychic (Gardner, 2001). FC's use was lauded as a breakthrough and educators and therapists could finally access the thoughts and feelings of individuals who were claimed to be "trapped" within their own bodies. The media endorsed the adoption of FC and stories, movies, and television shows were developed and distributed. Despite the widespread appeal, FC had many skeptics who began investigating and researching its practice. It did not take long to root out the flaws in FC's methodology.

Initial suspicion of FC arose when children receiving FC were observed looking away from the keyboard during sessions and failing to attend to activities (Gardner, 2001). A primary criticism of FC focuses on the authorship of the text produced by individuals participating in FC. Specifically, it was unknown whether individuals were authentically communicating through typing aided by facilitators. This was partially answered when a series of experimental studies demonstrating that the adult facilitators themselves were actually the ones directing the typing and the communication (see Green, 1994 for review). Researchers set up experiments whereby the individuals with ASD and their facilitators were blinded to one another's information to be typed (e.g., labeling pictures, responding to questions, describing activities). Participants always typed what facilitators saw, regardless of whether what they saw was the same as or different from the facilitator. Other studies found that when researchers asked individuals with ASD to respond to a simple question, responses were always incorrect or absent when facilitators did not know the question. Although Biklen et al. (1995) asserted that different responses produced across individuals who used FC were evidence that the responses were authentic and not produced by a facilitator, the debate about the efficacy of FC ended in the scientific community when numerous studies demonstrated that the facilitators controlled the content of the messages produced (Jacobson et al., 1995).

FC has not been able to hold up to decades of scrutiny by the scientific community. Early concerns about its use focused on a lack of scientific rigor and poor descriptions of the techniques used by the facilitators (Dillion, 1993; Green & Shane, 1993; Prior & Cummins, 1992). Early descriptions of FC emphasized providing clients with physical support and guidance, which later expanded to emphasis on providing clients with emotional support, such as trust and confidence in their ability to communicate (Travers et al., 2014). The ambiguity and vague methodological details led one reviewer of early FC articles to state "nothing here resembles research" (Thompson, 1994, p. 671). Proponents of FC have argued that controlled experimentation of FC invalidates it because it is confrontational in nature and destroys the participants' confidence (DEAL Communication Center, 1992). Despite claims that FC has results with valid outcomes, subsequent examination of FC methodology reveals significant flaws in design, observation, and measurement, rendering those outcomes questionable and dubious at best.

The central question to FC's utility and functionality as means for individuals with disabilities to communicate is whether the authorship of the messages is truly theirs. Immediately after FC was introduced, questions arose on the validity of the messages produced because of the role of the facilitator in their production (Silliman, 1992). That is, what role did a facilitator play in the production of messages? Furthermore, additional questions emerged on the reliance of FC to evoke communication consistently and across a range of situations and contexts, as would be required in one's typical environment. Could one produce messages with different facilitators, about different topics and situations (novel and familiar), across a variety of environments, over time? Numerous controlled investigations have revealed that there is no evidence that FC enables individuals to communicate reliably or effectively and the role of the facilitator in producing any appreciable communication cannot be ruled out (see Green & Shane, 1994 for further discussion). To be fair, many, if not most facilitators, were not acting in bad faith. They likely believed they were helping provide augmentative communication, and they were unconsciously deceiving themselves by way of the *ideomotor effect* (which is also how Ouija boards often work as well).

The harms associated with FC are well documented in the professional literature and over 20 professional organizations (e.g., American Academy of Child and Adolescent Psychiatry, American Academy of Pediatrics, American Psychological Association, American Speech-Language Hearing Association). Both governmental entities (e.g., New York State Department of Health, New Zealand Ministries of Health and Education) and professional organizations have released resolutions against the use of FC (Behavior Analysis Association of Michigan, 2022). For example, numerous allegations have been made through FC accusing caregivers, family members, and school and program personnel of abusive behavior, often sexual in nature. Many of these allegations were eventually proven to be false (Ganz, 2014). In addition, FC might be portrayed as a form of manipulation. Green (1994) described FC as a "somewhat unusual kind of abuse: allowing others to impose their own wishes, fears, hopes, and agendas on nonspeaking individuals" (p. 71). Finally, FC promotes dependence on another person for communication and perpetuates the myth that individuals with disabilities cannot learn to communicate independently (i.e., "dependence, disguised as advocacy," p. 198; Travers et al., 2014). Proponents of FC argue that its use is an augmentative and alternative communication (AAC) technique, but genuine, evidence-based interventions seek to teach independent communication, something FC has never been able to do as it has always required the use of a facilitator.

Summary and Conclusion

Pseudoscientific practices have gained acceptance within the educational community despite the dearth of any substantive scientific validation of these practices. Parents, educators, and caregivers have succumbed to the promise of improvement over measured outcomes, under the guise of treatment. SIT often uses obfuscated research methodology, subjective outcome measures, and poorly described procedures to claim effectiveness in treating hypothetical centralized deficits. AIT suffers from a dearth of high-quality research, subjective outcome measures, and is not recommended by several reputable professional organizations. FC is especially cruel as its proponents deceive parents and caregivers into believing that the typed messages are from the person with the neurodevelopmental disorder, when much research has demonstrated that it is the facilitator who is the one creating the messages.

Practitioners have much to do to overcome the attraction to and practice of pseudoscientific approaches in the treatment of individuals with neurodevelopmental disabilities. "When professionals and families approach intervention decisions buoyed by emotion rather than reason, optimism rather than skepticism, and anecdote rather than data, they ultimately become victims of an industry preying on benevolent but desperate people behaving under duress" (Travers et al., 2016, p. 287). Until practitioners embrace a more critical approach to the treatment of neurodevelopmental disorders, the "treatments" outlined in this discussion will continue to be used, depriving a vulnerable population of effective interventions that will serve to improve their independence and quality of life.

References

Addison, L. R., Piazza, C. C., Patel, M. R., Bachmeyer, M. H., Rivas, K. M., Milnes, S. M., & Oddo, J. (2012). A comparison of sensory integrative and behavioral therapies as treatment for pediatric feeding disorders. *Journal of Applied Behavior Analysis*, 45(3), 455–471. 10.1901/jaba.2012.45-455

Al-Ayadhi, L., Alhowikan, A. M., & Halepoto, D. M. (2018). Impact of auditory integrative training on transforming growth factor-β1 and its effect on behavioral and social emotions in children with autism spectrum disorder. *Medical Principles and Practice*, 27(1), 23–29. 10.1159/000486572

Al-Ayadhi, L., El-Ansary, A., Bjørklund, G., Chirumbolo, S., & Mostafa, G. A. (2019). Impact of auditory integration therapy (AIT) on the plasma levels of human glial cell line-derived neurotrophic factor (GDNF) in autism spectrum disorder. *The Journal of Molecular Neuroscience*, 68(4), 688–695. 10.1007/s12031-019-01332-w

American Academy of Pediatrics. (1998). Auditory integration training and facilitated communication for autism. American Academy of Pediatrics. Committee on Children with Disabilities. *Pediatrics*, 102(2 Pt 1), 431–433.

American Speech-Language Hearing Association (2004). *Auditory Integration Training*. Retrieved 04/21/2022 from https://www.asha.org/policy/tr2004-00260/

Andelin, L., Reynolds, S., & Schoen, S. (2021). Effectiveness of occupational therapy using a sensory integration approach: A multiple-baseline design study. *The American Journal of Occupational Therapy*, 75(6). 10.5014/ajot.2021.044917

Ashburner, J. K., Rodger, S. A., Ziviani, J. M., & Hinder, E. A. (2014). Comment on: 'An Intervention for Sensory Difficulties in Children with Autism: A Randomized Trial' by Schaaf et al. (2013). *Journal of Autism and Developmental Disorders*, 44(6), 1486–1488. 10.1007/s10803-014-2083-0

Baranek, G. T. (2002). Efficacy of sensory and motor interventions for children with autism. *Journal of Autism and Developmental Disorders*, 32(5), 397–422. 10.1023/A:1020541906063

Behavior Analysis Association of Michigan.(2022). *Resolutions and statements by scientific, professional, medical, governmental, and support organizations against the use of facilitated communication. Facilitated communication.*. http://baam. emich.edu/baam-fc-resolutions-compilation.html.

Berkell, D. E., Malgeri, S. E., & Streit, M. K. (1996). Auditory integration training for individuals with autism. *Education & Training in Mental Retardation & Developmental Disabilities*, 31(1), 66–70.

Bettison, S. (1996). The long-term effects of auditory training on children with autism. *Journal of Autism and Developmental Disorders, 26,* 361–374.

Biklen, D. (1990). Communication unbound: Autism and praxis. *Harvard Educational Review, 60*(3), 291–314. 10.17763/haer.60.3.013h5022862vu732

Biklen, D. (1993). *Communication unbound: How facilitated communication is challenging traditional views of autism and ability/disability. Special Education Series #13.* Teachers College Press, Columbia University.

Biklen, D., Morton, M. W., Gold, D., Berrigan, C., & Swaminathan, S. (1992). Facilitated communication: Implications for individuals with autism. *Topics in language disorders, 12*(4), 1.

Biklen, D., Saha, N., & Kliewer, C. (1995). How teachers confirm the authorship of facilitated communication: A portfolio approach. *Journal of the Association for Persons with Severe Handicaps, 20*(1), 45.

Biklen, D., & Schubert, A. (1991). New words: The communication of students with autism. *Remedial and Special Education, 12*(6), 46–57. 10.1177/07419325 9101200607

Brown, M. M. (1999). Auditory integration training and autism: Two case studies [case study]. *British Journal of Occupational Therapy, 62*(1), 13–18.

Camarata, S., Miller, L. J., & Wallace, M. T. (2020). Evaluating sensory integration/sensory processing treatment: Issues and analysis. *Frontiers in Integrative Neuroscience, 14.* 10.3389/fnint.2020.556660

Clark, G. F., Watling, R., Parham, L. D., & Schaaf, R. (2019). Occupational therapy interventions for children and youth with challenges in sensory integration and sensory processing: A school-based practice case example. *The American Journal of Occupational Therapy, 73*(3), 7303390010p7303390011–7303390010p730 3390018. 10.5014/ajot.2019.733001

Crossley, R., & McDonald, A. (1980). *Annie's coming out.* Penguin Books.

Davis, T. N., Durand, S., & Chan, J. M. (2011). The effects of a brushing procedure on stereotypical behavior. *Research in Autism Spectrum Disorders, 5*(3), 1053–1058. 10.1016/j.rasd.2010.11.011

Dawson, G., & Watling, R. (2000). Interventions to facilitate auditory, visual, and motor integration in autism: A review of the evidence. *Journal of Autism and Developmental Disorders, 30*(5), 415–421. 10.1023/A:1005547422749 (Treatments for people with autism and other pervasive developmental disorders: Research perspectives)

DEAL Communication Center (1992). *Facilitated Communication Training.*

Dillion, K. M. (1993). Facilitated communication, autism, and ouija. (includes related articles). *17*(3), 281–287.

Duchan, J. F. (1993). Issues raised by facilitated communication for theorizing and research on autism. *Journal of speech and hearing research, 36*(6), 1108–1119.

Edelson, S. M., Arin, D., Bauman, M., Lukas, S. E., Rudy, J. H., Sholar, M., & Rimland, B. (1999). Auditory integration training: A double-blind study of behavioral and electrophysiological effects in people with autism. *Focus on Autism and Other Developmental Disabilities, 14*(2), 73–81. 10.1177/108835 769901400202

Fazlioğlu, Y., & Baran, G. (2008). A sensory integration therapy program on sensory problems for children with autism. *Perceptual and Motor Skills, 106*(2), 415–422. 10.2466/pms.106.2.415-422

Ganz, J. B. (2014). The controversy surrounding facilitated communication. *Aided Augmentative Communication for Individuals with Autism Spectrum Disorders,* Springer. 115–126.

Gardner, M. (2001). Facilitated communication: A cruel farce. *Skeptical Inquirer, 25*(1), 17–19.

Gillberg, C., Johansson, M., Steffenburg, S., & Berlin, O. (1997). Auditory integration training in children with autism: Brief report of an open pilot study. *Autism: The International Journal of Research and Practice, 1*(1), 97–100. 10.1177/1362361397011009

Gillberg, C., Johansson, M., Steffenburg, S., & Berlin, Ö. (1998). 'Auditory integration training in children with autism': Reply to Rimland and Edelson. *Autism, 2*(1), 93–94. 10.1177/1362361398021010

Goldstein, H. (2000). Commentary: Interventions to facilitate auditory, visual, and motor integration: 'Show me the data'. *Journal of Autism and Developmental Disorders, 30*(5), 423–425. 10.1023/A:1005599406819 (Treatments for people with autism and other pervasive developmental disorders: Research perspectives)

Goldstein, H. (2003). Response to Edelson, Rimland, and Grandin's commentary. *Journal of Autism and Developmental Disorders, 33*(5), 553–555. 10.1023/A: 1025895915605

Gravel, J. S. (1994). Auditory integration training: Placing the burden of proof. *American Journal of Speech-language Pathology, 3*(2), 25–29.

Green, G. (1994). Facilitated communication: Mental miracle or sleight of hand? *Behavior and Social Issues, 4*(1-2), 69–85.

Green, G. (1996). Evaluating claims about treatments for autism. In C. Maurice, G. Green, & S. C. Luce (Eds.), *Behavioral intervention for young children with autism: A manual for parents and professionals* (pp. 15–28). PRO-ED.

Green, G., & Shane, H. C. (1993). Facilitated communication: The claims vs. the evidence. *Harvard Mental Health Letter, 10,* 4–5.

Green, G., & Shane, H. C. (1994). Science, reason, and facilitated communication. *Journal of the Association for Persons with Severe Handicaps, 19*(3), 151.

Green, V. A., Pituch, K. A., Itchon, J., Choi, A., O'Reilly, M., & Sigafoos, J. (2006). Internet survey of treatments used by parents of children with autism. *Research in Developmental Disabilities, 27*(1), 70–84. 10.1016/j.ridd.2004. 12.002

Howlin, P. (1997). When is a significant change not significant?. *Journal of Autism and Developmental Disorders, 27*(3), 347–348.

Iwanaga, R., Honda, S., Nakane, H., Tanaka, K., Toeda, H., & Tanaka, G. (2014). Pilot study: Efficacy of sensory integration therapy for Japanese children with high-functioning autism spectrum disorder: Sensory integration therapy for ASD. *Occupational Therapy International, 21*(1), 4–11. 10.1002/oti.1357

Jacobson, J. W., Foxx, R. M., & Mulick, J. A. (2015). Facilitated communication: The ultimate fad treatment. In R. M. Foxx & J. A. Mulick (Eds.), *Controversial therapies for autism and intellectual disabilities* (pp. 283–302). Routledge.

Jacobson, J. W., Mulick, J. A., & Schwartz, A. A. (1995). A history of facilitated communication: science, pseudoscience, and antiscience. *The American Psychologist, 50*(9), 750–765.

Kashefimehr, B., Kayihan, H., & Huri, M. (2018). The effect of sensory integration therapy on occupational performance in children with autism. *OTJR, 38*(2), 75–83. 10.1177/1539449217743456

Ledbetter-Cho, K., Lang, R., Davenport, K., Moore, M., Lee, A., Howell, A., Drew, C., Dawson, D., Charlop, M. H., Falcomata, T., & O'Reilly, M. (2015). Effects of script training on the peer-to-peer communication of children with autism spectrum disorder. *Journal of Applied Behavior Analysis, 48*(4), 785–799. 10.1002/jaba.240

Link, H. M. (1997). Auditory Integration Training (AIT): Sound therapy? Case studies of three boys with autism who received AIT. *British Journal of Learning Disabilities, 25*(3), 106–110. 10.1111/j.1468-3156.1997.tb00021.x

Lydon, H., Healy, O., & Grey, I. (2017). Comparison of behavioral intervention and sensory integration therapy on challenging behavior of children with autism. *Behavioral Interventions, 32*(4), 297–310. 10.1002/bin.1490

Metz, B., Mulick, J. A., & Butter, E. M. (2015). Autism: A twenty-first century fad magnet. In R. M. Foxx & J. A. Mulick (Eds.), *Controversial therapies for autism and intellectual disabilities* (pp. 189–215). Routledge.

Mills, C. J., Michail, E., & Bye, R. A. (2020). A survey of occupational therapists on a new tool for sensory processing. *Occupational Therapy International, 2020.* 10.1155/2020/5909347

Mudford, O. C., Cross, B. A., Breen, S., Cullen, C., Reeves, D., Gould, J., & Douglas, J. (2000). Auditory integration training for children with autism: No behavioral benefits detected. *American Journal of Mental Retardation, 105*(2), 118–129. 10.1352/0895-8017(2000)105<0118:AITFCW>2.0.CO;2

Mudford, O. C., & Cullen, C. (2016). Auditory integration training: A critical review (1991–2014). In R. M. Foxx & J. A. Mulick (Eds.), *Controversial therapies for autism and intellectual disabilities: Fad, fashion, and science in professional practice* (2 ed., pp. 270–282). Routledge.

National Autism Center. (2015). *Findings and conclusions: National standards project, phase 2.*Randolph, MA: Author.

Omairi, C., Mailloux, Z., Antoniuk, S. A., & Schaaf, R. (2022). Occupational therapy using Ayres sensory integration®: A randomized controlled trial in Brazil. *Am J Occup Ther, 76*(4). 10.5014/ajot.2022.048249

Parham, L. D., Clark, G. F., Watling, R., & Schaaf, R. (2019). Occupational therapy interventions for children and youth with challenges in sensory integration and sensory processing: A clinic-based practice case example. *American Journal of Occupational Therapy, 73*(1), 1–9.

Parham, L. D., Roley, S. S., May-Benson, T. A., Koomar, J., Brett-Green, B., Burke, J. P., Cohn, E. S., Mailloux, Z., Miller, L. J., & Schaaf, R. C. (2011). Development of a fidelity measure for research on the effectiveness of the Ayres Sensory Integration intervention. *The American journal of occupational therapy, 65*(2), 133–142. 10.5014/ajot.2011.000745

Parr, J. (2010). Autism. *BMJ Clin Evid, 2010.*

Pfeiffer, B. A., Koenig, K., Kinnealey, M., Sheppard, M., & Henderson, L. (2011). Effectiveness of sensory integration interventions in children with autism spectrum disorders: a pilot study. *The American Journal of Occupational Therapy*, 65(1), 76–85. 10.5014/ajot.2011.09205

Prior, M., & Cummins, R. (1992). Questions about facilitated communication and autism. *Journal of Autism and Developmental Disorders*, 22(3), 331–337. 10.1007/BF01048237

Rimland, B., & Edelson, S. M. (1995). Brief report: A pilot study of auditory integration training in autism. *Journal of Autism and Developmental Disorders*, 25, 61–70.

Roberts, J. E., King-Thomas, L., & Boccia, M. L. (2007). Behavioral indexes of the efficacy of sensory integration therapy. *The American Journal of Occupational Therapy*, 61(5), 555–562. 10.5014/ajot.61.5.555

Roley, S. S. M., Zoe, Miller-Kuhanek, H., & Glennon, T. J. (2007). Understanding Ayres' sensory integration. *OT Practice* 12(17), 1–8.

Rossignol, D. (2009). Novel and emerging treatments for autism spectrum disorders: A systematic review. *Annals of Clinical Psychiatry*, 21(4), 213–236.

Schaaf, R., & Blanche, E. I. (2011). Comparison of behavioral intervention and sensory-integration therapy in the treatment of challenging behavior. *Journal of Autism and Developmental Disorders*, 41(10), 1436–1438. 10.1007/s10803-011-1303-0

Schaaf, R. C. (2011). Interventions that address sensory dysfunction for individuals with autism spectrum disorders: Preliminary evidence for the superiority of sensory integration compared to other sensory approaches. In B. Reichow, P. Doehring, D. V. Cicchetti, & F. R. Volkmar (Eds.), *Evidence-based practices and treatments for children with autism* (pp. 245–273). Springer Science + Business Media. 10.1007/978-1-4419-6975-0_9

Schaaf, R. C., Benevides, T., Mailloux, Z., Faller, P., Hunt, J., van Hooydonk, E., Freeman, R., Leiby, B., Sendecki, J., & Kelly, D. (2013). An intervention for sensory difficulties in children with autism: A randomized trial. *Journal of Autism and Developmental Disorders*, 44(7), 1493–1506. 10.1007/s10803-013-1983-8

Schaaf, R. C., Benevides, T. W., Kelly, D., & Mailloux-Maggio, Z. (2012). Occupational therapy and sensory integration for children with autism: A feasibility, safety, acceptability and fidelity study. *Autism*, 16(3), 321–327. 10.1177/1362361311435157

Schaaf, R. C., Dumont, R. L., Arbesman, M., & May-Benson, T. A. (2018). Efficacy of occupational therapy using Ayres sensory integration(®): A systematic review. *American Journal of Occupational Therapy*, 72(1), 7201190010p7201190011-7201190010p7201190010. 10.5014/ajot.2018.028431

Schoen, S. A., Schaaf, R. C., Mailloux, Z., Bundy, A., Lane, S., May-Benson, T. A., Parham, L. D., & Roley, S. S. (2022). Response: Commentary: Evaluating sensory integration/sensory processing treatment: Issues and analysis. *Frontiers in Integrative Neuroscience*, 16. 10.3389/fnint.2022.874320

Schreck, K. A. (2014). Parents and autism treatment choices. In V. B. Patel & C. R. Martin (Eds.), *A comprehensive guide to autism* (pp. 2283–2296).

Siegel, B., & Zimnitzky, B. (1998). Assessing 'alternative' therapies for communication disorders in children with autistic spectrum disorders: Facilitated communication and auditory integration training. *Journal of Speech-language Pathology and Audiology, 22*(2), 61–70.

Silliman, E. R. (1992). Three perspectives of facilitated communication: Unexpected literacy, Clever Hans, or enigma?. *Topics in Language Disorders, 12*(4), 60–68.

Sinha, Y., Silove, N., Hayen, A., & Williams, K. (2011). Auditory integration training and other sound therapies for autism spectrum disorders (ASD). *Cochrane Database of Systematic Reviews,* (12), CD003681. 10.1002/14651 858.CD003681.pub3

Smith, T., Mruzek, D. W., & Mozingo, D. B. (2016). Sensory integration therapy. In R. M. Foxx & J. A. Mulick (Eds.), *Controversial therapies for autism and intellectual disabilities* (2 ed., pp. 246–268). 10.4324/9781315754345-15

Sokhadze, E. M., Casanova, M. F., Tasman, A., & Brockett, S. (2016). Electrophysiological and behavioral outcomes of berard auditory integration training (AIT) in children with autism spectrum disorder. *Applied Psychophysiology and Biofeedback, 41*(4), 405–420. 10.1007/s10484-016-9343-z

Stevenson, B. S. (2019). Response to 'Application of the Council for Exceptional Children's Standards for Evidence-Based Practices in Special Education' by Schoen et al [2019]. *Autism Research, 12*(8), 1152–1153. 10.1002/aur.2165

Tharpe, A. M. (1999). Auditory integration training: The magical mystery cure. *Language, Speech & Hearing Services in Schools, 30*(4), 378–382. 10.1044/0161-1461.3004.378

Thompson, T. (1994). Review of communication unbound by Douglas Biklen. *American Journal of Mental Retardation, 98,* 670–673.

Travers, J. C., Tincani, M. J., & Lang, R. (2014). Facilitated communication denies people with disabilities their voice. *Research and Practice for Persons with Severe Disabilities, 39*(3), 195–202. 10.1177/1540796914556778

Travers, J. C., Ayers, K., Simpson, R. L., & Crutchfield, S. (2016). Fad, Pseudoscientific, and controversial interventions, *Evidence-based practices in behavioral health, early intervention for young children with autism spectrum disorder* (pp. 257–293).

Watkins, N., & Sparling, E. (2014). The effectiveness of the Snug Vest on stereotypic behaviors in children diagnosed with an autism spectrum disorder. *Behavior Modification, 38*(3), 412–427. 10.1177/0145445514532128

Williames, L. D., & Erdie-Lalena, C. R. (2009). Complementary, holistic, and integrative medicine: sensory integration. *Pediatric Review, 30*(12), e91–e93. 10.1542/pir.30-12-e91

Zimmer, M., Desch, L., Rosen, L. D., Bailey, M. L., Becker, D., Culbert, T. P. … Wiley, S. E. (2012). Sensory integration therapies for children with developmental and behavioral disorders. Policy Statement from the American Academy of Pediatrics. *Pediatrics, 126,* 1186–1189.

13 Externalizing Behaviors

Maddison Knott, Arianna Delgadillo, Sara Jordan, Lauren Erp, and Audrey Ambrosio

Externalizing behaviors have been conceptualized as overt behavior problems, which include disruptive, hyperactive, and aggressive behaviors (Liu, 2004). Within school settings, externalizing behaviors, such as talking out of order, refusal to follow directions, and off-task behaviors, are common (Egger & Angold, 2006). For example, a study by Floress et al. (2018) demonstrated that preschool children engaged in externalizing behaviors during approximately 14% of the observation intervals across general, at-risk, and special education classrooms. There is usually a decline in externalizing behaviors when children reach school age; however, for some these behaviors increase. The literature has shown that these behaviors can be associated with a host of negative outcomes for students, including academic difficulties, peer rejection, and poor personal adjustment (Baker et al., 2008; Samek & Hicks, 2014). In addition, students with externalizing behaviors demand attention from teachers and disrupt the learning environment for others (Lassen et al., 2006). Moreover, managing externalizing behaviors is a major source of teacher stress (Boudreault & Lessard, 2020).

Various behavior management practices have been used in schools to help prevent or reduce externalizing behaviors, including positive reinforcement, punishment, and antecedent-based approaches (Clunies-Ross et al., 2008; O'Connor & Hayes, 2020). These interventions have been developed based largely on operant learning theory which posits that disruptive behaviors in the classroom stem from a history of reinforcement of those behaviors under certain stimulus conditions. However, some researchers purport that reinforcement or punishment may influence the students' behavior by altering their motivation to engage in tasks or behavior appropriately (Clunies-Ross et al., 2008; O'Connor & Hayes, 2020; Reeve, 2012).

To address externalizing behavior problems in school settings, some school professionals have been hesitant to utilize techniques rooted in behaviorism that involve rewarding appropriate and penalizing

DOI: 10.4324/9781003266181-18

inappropriate student behaviors. As such, this chapter will investigate two primary claims: 1) intrinsic motivation is better than extrinsic motivation, and 2) external rewards undermine intrinsic motivation.

Examining the Claims

Alfie Kohn (1993) infers from hundreds of studies to convey how incentives such as rewards, gold stars, praise, and punishments impede students' ability to learn from their experiences and may lessen their motivation to produce desirable responses in the future. Some school professionals have also challenged the use of external rewards and have claimed that interventions fostering intrinsic motivation, or the personal interest to self-manage behavior, is the best method to reduce externalizing behaviors (Deci & Ryan, 1985). Theories of motivation have contributed to long and important debates regarding the best practices associated with working with students' problem behavior. Given the prevalence and impact of externalizing behaviors in classrooms, it is important to discuss evidence-based practices and the role of motivation in the management of externalizing behaviors.

Claim #1: Intrinsic Motivation Is Better than Extrinsic Motivation

Motivation has been defined as a force that produces a desire for a goal and directs behavior in a particular direction to achieve a goal (Kong, 2009). Social-cognitive theorists have identified two distinct types of motivation: intrinsic motivation and extrinsic motivation (Ryan & Deci, 2000). Intrinsic motivation attributes behavioral outcomes to internal processes, whereas extrinsic motivation attributes behavioral outcomes to external sources of reinforcement and punishment. An example of an intrinsically motivated behavior would be an individual reading because of the simple enjoyment of reading, not because their reading behavior has been previously rewarded through reinforcers such as praise or free personal pan pizzas (Deci & Ryan, 1985). These researchers claim that intrinsically motivated behaviors are natural responses to an environment's structure or occur "by default" (Deci & Ryan, 1985; Zimmerman, 1985). By contrast, extrinsic motivation is characterized by behaviors that are programmed by others, such as parents or teachers through use of external rewards (Deci & Ryan, 1985). Simply stated, students who engage in behaviors to receive a reward or avoid a punishment are considered to be extrinsically motivated, whereas students who choose to do so for personal satisfaction, knowledge, or achievement are said to be intrinsically motivated (Serin, 2018). It is a commonly held belief in school settings that intrinsic motivation is superior to extrinsic motivation.

Self-determination theory (SDT; Deci & Ryan, 1985) suggests that people are naturally driven to acquire the psychological skills of autonomy, competency, and relatedness (Deci & Ryan, 1985, 1991). According to SDT researchers, students are more likely to display self-determined (i.e., autonomous) behavior (Guay, 2021; Tian et al., 2018) when their psychological needs are met. For example, a self-determined student would believe that their behaviors are of their own volition (i.e., autonomous) and are chosen so that they can interact effectively in their environment (i.e., competence) and feel connected to their teachers and peers (i.e., relatedness). Fousiani (2011) theorized that when autonomy, competency, and relatedness are not fully developed, students may feel that their compliance was not of their own volition, but instead due to external pressure to behave in a certain way. As a result, students may feel a lack of control in their lives and present as noncompliant, defiant, and disengaged (Guay, 2021; Ryan et al., 2021). Together, SDT researchers have used research findings to claim that motivation alone drives behavior.

When SDT was first developed, studies focused on the dichotomy between extrinsic and intrinsic motivation. While external motivators were shown to effectively change behavior in the short term (Wilson & Corpus, 2001), researchers claimed that intrinsic motivators were associated with higher-quality motivation that was more effective in the long term (Ryan & Deci, 2000a). Indeed, a longitudinal study examining the effects of different motivation types on academic achievement found that intrinsic motivation was not only a stronger predictor than extrinsic reinforcement, but it was also the only factor that consistently predicted achievement across time (Taylor et al., 2014). Findings similar to these led researchers and other professionals to question and eventually undermine the practical value of extrinsic motivation in educational contexts. Thus, early frameworks of SDT may have contributed to research and practices that have disparaged feasible options to decrease frequency of externalizing behaviors in schools.

Claim #2 External Rewards Undermine Intrinsic Motivation

The over justification hypothesis (OJH) theorizes that external rewards have a negative impact on students' natural or intrinsic motivation to learn and complete tasks. First introduced by Deci (1971), the OJH suggests that external rewards are harmful because once provided, students will no longer complete the task without external rewards. Additionally, these rewards must be increased over time in order to maintain the behavior. Thus, the OJH concludes that external rewards have a detrimental impact on one's intrinsic desire and interest to engage in desired behaviors (Deci, 1971; Guay et al., 2021; Lepper et al., 1973).

The OJH followed from self-perception theory which suggests that individuals believe that they are intrinsically motivated to perform an action or engage in an activity if they do not perceive or receive extrinsic consequences (i.e., rewards) to which they can attribute their behavior (Bem, 1965; Kelley, 1973). In other words, if an individual does not initially perceive their engagement in certain behaviors as solely based on receiving an external reward, then they are more likely to maintain their intrinsic motivation. Consequently, the individual, who was initially intrinsically motivated to engage in a certain behavior, is now less likely to be intrinsically motivated toward that behavior after having received an extrinsic reward. The rewarded individual may now come to infer that their actions were solely motivated by the external reward rather than the activity itself. Therefore, the individual no longer sees the activity as an end in itself (Lepper, 1973).

The literature has also used this hypothesis as evidence that extrinsic motivators are not effective in the long term and that they may cause harm to an individual's reward system, especially if the extrinsic reward is removed. For example, Deci (1971) presented the example of a child who mows the lawn. The child may start out mowing the lawn because he enjoys the activity, but he begins receiving compensation for his efforts from neighbors and friends. Deci (1971) hypothesized that the child will eventually attribute his enjoyment of mowing the lawn to receiving compensation. Therefore, he may eventually not enjoy mowing the lawn, if he no longer receives compensation for his efforts. Therefore, the child will be less likely to engage in the activity on his own out of pure enjoyment.

Lepper et al. (1973) was one of the first studies that supported the originally proposed OJH by Deci (1971). Lepper et al. (1973) sought to observe the effects of extrinsic rewards on preschool children's intrinsic motivation to draw. Intrinsic "interest" in drawing was operationally defined as the percentage of time the child spent sitting at a table with drawing materials or placing a hand on a magic marker. The results of their observations showed that children who were expecting to receive a reward showed less intrinsic interest in drawing compared to students who were not expecting a reward. The researchers concluded that intrinsic motivation to complete the task was reduced among rewarded children and their performances were over justified. According to the hypothesis, the children's intrinsic motivation was diminished by the experience of being rewarded for a behavior they used to engage in without extrinsic reward. Therefore, children may not willingly engage in future similar tasks in the absence of a reward. In other words, they may believe that they are only completing the task to receive a reward. Many later motivation researchers have had the same concerns and have found similar results in their studies.

For example, Gneezy and Rustichini (2000) sought to examine the effects that compensation had on high school students who were asked to collect money for a charity event. Their results again supported the claims of the OJH in which high schoolers collected more money and showed more effort in collecting donations when no compensation was given compared to students who received compensation. Therefore, the researchers concluded that students who were compensated showed less intrinsic motivation and less effort, further confirming this belief in negative effects of external rewards for desired behavior.

These results further inform the effects the OJH may have in academic settings. Teachers have previously rewarded students for their performance, be it finishing tasks or displaying exemplary behavior. However, Gneezy et al. (2011) purported that offering rewards to improve academic performance may provide students with several possible perspectives about their motivation and performance: (a) The task is difficult, (b) the task is not attractive or interesting, (c) the student is not well-suited to accomplish the task, and/or (d) the teacher (or the rewarder) does not trust in the student's intrinsic motivation. Gneezy et al. (2011) further emphasized that such perspectives may have harmful effects on students' self-efficacy, confidence, and intrinsic motivation. Instead of encouraging students to engage in the task on their own merit, they may be discouraged and made to believe the perspectives noted above. Later researchers continued to support the OJH in which their findings determined that rewards were considered to be, at best, bribery (Kohn, 1993) and, at worst, a form of psychological control in which students feel obligated or guilted into behaving appropriately (Guay, 2022).

Deeper Dive into These Claims

Is intrinsic motivation better than extrinsic motivation? And if so, do external rewards actually undermine intrinsic motivation? Also, are measures of intrinsic motivation valid in that they measure what they intend to measure? To answer these questions, first we need to better understand what is meant by motivation. Akin-Little and Little (2019) describe many methodological and construct formation concerns with the social-cognitive perspectives of motivation. For example, social-cognitive researchers claim that intrinsic motivation strictly does not form based on external reinforcers and that decrease of intrinsic motivation is due to use of external incentives to increase or sustain behaviors. However, previous research suggests that the decrease of "intrinsic motivation" may be due to other competing contingencies operating in the environment that consequently reinforce and maintain some behaviors and extinguish others (Flora, 1990; Reiss & Sushinsky, 1975).

Akin and Little (2019) explain that the results of studies attempting to measure intrinsic motivation may have misinterpretations of observed data. For example, Dickinson's (1989) study attempted to extrinsically reinforce intrinsically motivated activities, such as dance or painting. However, before the researcher began implementing extrinsic rewards, the individual often received verbal praise for engaging in the activity. When extrinsic rewards were introduced, the researcher stopped giving verbal praise. Expectedly, the individual was no longer as motivated to engage in the activity likely because they were not receiving praise, a previous reinforcement, as they had been before (Akin & Little, 2019). The authors interpreted this behavior change as a decline in intrinsic motivation. Many social-cognitive researchers would expect dance to be maintained by intrinsic motivation, but in this case, it is evident that dance was initially reinforced and maintained through use of external verbal praise. Indeed, findings from Cameron and Pierce's (1994) meta-analysis first pointed out that verbal praise and positive feedback are two of the main factors that influence intrinsic motivation.

Carton (1996) also brought to light methodological concerns in social-cognitive studies in which many external reinforcers were given days to weeks after participation in the treatment setting, whereas verbal rewards were given immediately. Therefore, the reduced impact of external reinforcers may have been due to the delay rather than the form of reward (Carton, 1996). Furthermore, another methodological short-coming concerns the reliability and construct validity of measures of intrinsic motivation (Reiss, 2005). Many cognitive theorists, such as Deci and Ryan (1985), provide no direct evidence to support their theories that attempt to explain the drive of intrinsic motivation. This is largely because there is no clearly agreed-upon operational definition of intrinsic motivation, thus, there is no psychometrically sound method of measuring intrinsic motivation. Absent a clear definition and means of measuring this construct, researchers have relied on making inferences that confirm their theory (Reiss, 2005) to interpret experimental findings. For example, when undermining effects of rewards were expected and observed by decrease in behavior, researchers inferred a reduction in intrinsic motivation. However, those studies that did not observe undermining effects in the extrinsically reinforced groups were dismissed (Reiss, 2005).

Due to the likely misinterpretations of findings on intrinsic motivation and flaws in methodology, it is clear why this topic is highly debated. Several meta-analyses and specific studies have been conducted to examine and conceptualize intrinsic and extrinsic motivation. However, meta-analyses have compiled studies that compared usages of intrinsic and extrinsic rewards and they found no detrimental effects of external reinforcement on intrinsic motivation (Cameron et al., 2001; Cameron & Pierce, 1994;

Workman & Williams, 1980). For example, Workman and Williams (1980) investigated the effects of rewards on intrinsic motivation in the classroom, specifically examining task behavior. Their results found that external reinforcement increased and maintained the students' task engagement in a number of studies involving follow-ups ranging from 2 to 5 days up to 12 months duration (Hall et al., 1968; Simmons & Wasik, 1973; Walker & Hops, 1976; Workman & Williams, 1980). Furthermore, the conclusions of Cameron and Pierce's (1994) meta-analysis revealed that rewards are generally not detrimental to intrinsic motivation. Rather, if a reward is offered, regardless of level of performance, then intrinsic motivation has been shown to decrease. Therefore, rewards must be given for meeting a specified standard, level of expectation, or for completing a task for desired behaviors to increase.

Motivational theories have highly influenced schools and their ways of managing students' behaviors. Some theorists hold firm to the OJH which claims that external rewards overcompensate for expected, appropriate behaviors, especially in the classroom. Furthermore, they claim that providing token systems, star charts, money, or promise of a bigger reward is over justifying student behaviors and therefore decreasing their intrinsic motivation to engage with the activity in the future (Deci, 1971; Guay et al., 2021; Kohn et al., 1999; Lepper et al., 1973). However, the results of Flora and Flora (1999) examined the effects of extrinsic reinforcement for reading during childhood on later reading habits of college students. The findings refute the over justification claims in which reinforcing children's behavior with an external reward did not increase or decrease the amount of reading. Furthermore, it also did not influence later self-reported intrinsic motivation for reading. In fact, extrinsic reinforcement seems to have set the stage for later continued interest in reading (Flora & Flora, 1999).

Overall, the very idea of intrinsic motivation rests on belief in a hypothetical construct and indirect observation of behavior that cannot be directly measured. In other words, we do not have a way to objectively measure intrinsic motivation in the first place, yet many studies that claim a reduction in intrinsic motivation (such as in the dance example above) infer this change solely on the basis of a change in behavior (in this case, dance). This is circular reasoning. If we can't objectively measure intrinsic motivation, how can we infer a change in that motivation? All we can directly measure is the amount of dance before and after providing an external reward. However, there may be many other explanations for this change in dance behavior that were not considered. In this example, the researchers neglected to note other factors that changed, namely, the removal of verbal praise. In other situations, there may be competing contingencies of reinforcement that impact a student's behavior, such as peer attention reinforcing disruptive behavior, that are more powerful or salient to the student than an external reward such as a trinket from the prize box for staying on task.

Similarly, the concept of intrinsic motivation can be conceptualized from a behavioral perspective as an activity for which there is naturally occurring reinforcement. In other words, the activity is intrinsically motivating because it produces some form of outcome or consequence that is in and of itself reinforcing (also sometimes referred to as an activity that is maintained by automatic reinforcement). It could be enjoyment associated with doing the task itself or a sense of accomplishment or pride in the work product or outcome.

We often use extrinsic incentives (or more arbitrary/unnatural rewards like prizes, tokens, or money) to bridge and motivate students to engage in tasks until we reach a point wherein the tasks themselves (e.g., pride in making a good grade) become reinforcing in and of themselves. Extrinsic rewards are most likely to be needed when there is high response effort required or a task is difficult, a child is unlikely to be successful during initial efforts (e.g., learning a new skill), the outcomes of an action are delayed, or the child is not motivated by the same "intrinsic factors" as other children.

By reframing these concepts, there may very well be a kernel of truth to the notion that intrinsically motivated behaviors are preferable to extrinsically motivated behaviors. The ultimate goal of a successful intervention is that students do not have to rely on external incentives or other artificial forms of reinforcement indefinitely. Rather, it is preferred that external reinforcers be gradually spaced out and reduced and that appropriate behavior come under the control of more natural or internal sources of reinforcement such as social approval, pride, or sense of accomplishment. This is often achieved through use of fading and variable reinforcement schedules in order to reduce use of artificial reinforcers while maintaining the desired behavior. Nevertheless, the notion that external rewards undermine intrinsic motivation remains a point of disagreement among behavioral and social-cognitive researchers, although as we've shown, the studies that are foundational to these claims may not be as grounded in science as previously thought.

Potential Harms of Motivational Theories

Previous research has examined the effects of external rewards on intrinsic motivation, specifically regarding effects on externalizing behaviors in the classroom. These studies have provided evidence that external rewards are not detrimental to intrinsic motivation in regard to engagement in activities and completion of tasks. However, research has also had consistent findings when examining the effects of rewards on appropriate classroom behaviors. Akin-Little and Little (2004) examined over justification effects of a token economy for appropriate classroom behavior in a classroom setting. In this study, children were awarded tokens for appropriate behavior. If they acquired a certain number of tokens, they were provided a prize. The study found no over justification effect for any of the students. Instead, focusing attention on a student's current level of functioning, and how to deliver reinforcers based on observable, measurable criteria has been shown to be useful for both performance and acquisition deficits (Akin et al., 2004; Northup et al., 1996). Additionally, giving rewards for tasks that students find particularly difficult has been shown to "improve their motivation" (or likelihood of engaging in the task), meaning students were more likely to complete difficult tasks when offered rewards (Akin et al., 2004).

The OJH challenges the use of contingent rewards and has promoted dubious practices in schools. Teachers and other school personnel are basing their methods of managing externalizing behaviors in the classroom by relying on research findings that claim to measure intrinsic motivation. However, we do not have a way to objectively measure intrinsic or extrinsic motivation outside of the outcomes of a task (the child either engages in the task or does not). The belief that students will engage in certain behaviors purely due to their own intrinsic motivation is a potentially harmful perspective and will likely result in a lack of change in behavior or performance (Akin et al., 2004). This is particularly concerning when considering teaching students new skills or designing interventions for students with disabilities.

While some educators report that all rewards are harmful to students' motivation, the only detrimental effects that have been found on motivation were when the rewards were not explicitly connected to a task (Cameron et al., 2001). Teachers often set standards for student performance that the student cannot reach which results in no reward for their effort. This sends a message to the student that they have failed and may therefore lead to discouragement and what may be interpreted as a further decrease in motivation (Akin et al., 2004; Cameron et al., 2001). This is not surprising from a behavioral perspective because when a goal is too high and the student cannot reach it, their behavior then is never reinforced and is effectively on extinction. Therefore, desired behaviors and/or performance from the student are reduced. While some school personnel disagree with the use of extrinsic motivators despite frequent requests for behavior and classroom management technique training from teachers and studies that show the positive effects of rewards, Axelrod (1996) suggests that the resistance to this research may be due to rewards requiring too much time and removing free choice for students.

In other words, teachers may have the perspective that rewards are bribing a student to behave a certain way or engage in an activity instead of choosing to do so themselves. Overall, research has shown that relying solely on a student's intrinsic motivation for change and not providing extrinsic motivators can be ineffective, and potentially harmful to students.

Evidence-Based Practices for Management of Behavioral Concerns

Decades of research in the classroom have yielded a body of empirical literature with robust scientific evidence to support the efficacy of class-wide and individual student behavior management strategies. Among these evidence-based practices are interventions based on antecedent and consequence strategies such as schoolwide use of Positive Behavior Interventions and Supports (PBIS; Kim et al., 2018). PBIS encompasses a range of strategies and components, including classwide or individual contingency management approaches, such as the use of behavior-specific praise, token economies (Maggin et al., 2011), group contingency management techniques (i.e., the Good Behavior Game [Smith et al., 2021], Mystery Motivator [Kowalewicz & Coffee, 2014]) (Maggin et al., 2012), the Daily Behavior Report Card (Vannest, Davis, Mason & Burke), and Check In Check Out (Drevon et al., 2019), to name a few (see Riden et al., 2022 for a thorough compilation of meta-analyses and systematic reviews). Many of these evidence-based practices rely heavily on use of external reinforcement as a mechanism for reducing student externalizing behaviors. At the same time, there is little solid evidence that use of these strategies undermines students' intrinsic motivation to behave appropriately. Moreover, there is ample evidence that behavior change can be directly measured through observation and that the theoretical concept of motivation does not need to be invoked in order to address classroom behavioral concerns. As a result, educators need not be fearful of using incentives and rewards to improve student behavior.

Summary and Conclusion

This chapter discussed how motivation is multifaceted and cannot be objectively measured. Furthermore, inferring which facets of motivation are occurring to drive behavior is not reliable. Motivational and behavioral theories seek to understand and change behavior; however, motivational theories may bring us further away from uncovering what truly drives behavior. From a social-cognitive perspective, motivation is at the forefront of what needs to change before behavior will change. On the other hand, behaviorists seek to change behavior first and determine what interventions could aid in changing behavior. Many evidence-based practices focus on antecedents and consequences that reliably promote positive behaviors and discourage problem behaviors. School resources should be allocated appropriately to evidence-based practices that change behavior.

In short, it is important to recognize that external reinforcers play a crucial role in teaching school-aged children behavior management skills. The use of external reinforcers does not equate to bribing or undermining intrinsic motivation. Instead, it helps students establish a connection between their actions and positive outcomes. By reinforcing appropriate behaviors, we create opportunities for students to experience the inherent satisfaction and fulfillment that can come from engaging in those behaviors. Moreover, the real world operates on a system of external rewards and consequences. Few adults, for example, maintain a well-kept lawn because they are internally motivated. Rather, they are rewarded (or incentivized) with having a pleasant environment for family activities or by the desire to avoid complaints from neighbors. By introducing students to external reinforcers in a controlled educational setting, we are preparing them to navigate the larger world where such consequences naturally occur.

References

Akin-Little, K. A., Eckert, T. L., Lovett, B. J., & Little, S. G. (2004). Extrinsic reinforcement in the classroom: Bribery or best practice. *School Psychology Review*, *33*(3), 344–362.

Akin-Little, A., & Little, S. G. (2019). Effect of extrinsic reinforcement on "intrinsic" motivation: Separating fact from fiction. In S. G. Little & A. Akin-Little (Eds.), *Behavioral interventions in schools: Evidence-based positive strategies* (pp. 113–132), American Psychological Association.

Axelrod, S. (1996). What's wrong with behavior analysis?. *Journal of Behavioral Education*, *6*, 247–256.

Baker, J. A., Grant, S., & Morlock, L. (2008). The teacher-student relationship as a developmental context for children with internalizing or externalizing behavior problems. *School Psychology Quarterly*, *23*(1), 3–15.

Bem, D. J., Wallach, M. A., & Kogan, N. (1965). Group decision making under risk of aversive consequences. *Journal of Personality and Social Psychology*, *1*(5), 453.

Boudreault, A., & Lessard, J. (2020). Helping teachers manage students' externalizing behaviors by identifying behavioral cusps. *Canadian Journal for New Scholars in Education/Revue Canadienne des Jeunes Chercheures et Chercheurs en éducation*, *11*(1), 69–78.

Cameron, J., & Pierce, W. D. (1994). Reinforcement, reward, and intrinsic motivation: A meta-analysis. *Review of Educational Research*, *64*(3), 363–423.

Cameron, J., Banko, K. M., & Pierce, W. D. (2001). Pervasive negative effects of rewards on intrinsic motivation: The myth continues. *The Behavior Analyst*, *24*(1), 1–44.

Carton, J. S. (1996). The differential effects of tangible rewards and praise on intrinsic motivation: A comparison of cognitive evaluation theory and operant theory. *The Behavior Analyst, 19*, 237–255.

Clunies-Ross, P., Little, E., & Kienhuis, M. (2008). Self-reported and actual use of proactive and reactive classroom management strategies and their relationship with teacher stress and student behaviour. *Educational Psychology, 28*(6), 693–710.

Deci, E. L. (1971). Effects of externally mediated rewards on intrinsic motivation. *Journal of Personality and Social Psychology, 18*(1), 105.

Deci, E.,& Ryan, R. (1985). *Intrinsic motivation and self determination in human behavior.* NewYork: Plenum.

Deci, E. L., & Ryan, R. M. (1991). A motivational approach to self: Integration in personality. In R. A. Dienstbier (Ed.), *Nebraska Symposium on Motivation, 1990: Perspectives on motivation* (pp. 237–288). University of Nebraska Press.

Dickinson, A. M. (1989). The detrimental effects of extrinsic reinforcement on "intrinsic motivation". *The Behavior Analyst, 12*, 1–15.

Drevon, D. D., Hixson, M. D., Wyse, R. D., & Rigney, A. M. (2019). A meta-analytic review of the evidence for check-in check-out. *Psychology in the Schools, 56*(3), 393–412.

Egger, H. L., & Angold, A. (2006). Common emotional and behavioral disorders in preschool children: Presentation, nosology, and epidemiology. *Journal of Child Psychology and Psychiatry, 47*(3–4), 313–337.

Flora, S. R. (1990). Undermining intrinsic interest from the standpoint of a behaviorist. *The Psychological Record, 40*, 323–346.

Flora, S. R., & Flora, D. B. (1999). Effects of extrinsic reinforcement for reading during childhood on reported reading habits of college students. *The Psychological Record, 49*, 3–14.

Floress, M. T., Rader, R. A., Berlinghof, J. R., & Fanok, P. C. (2018). Externalizing behaviors within general, at-risk, and special education preschool classrooms: A preliminary investigation. *Preventing School Failure: Alternative Education for Children and Youth, 62*(4), 279–288.

Fousiani, K., Sakalaki, M., & Richardson, C. (2011). Opportunistic propensity hinders commitment to acts in conditions of forced compliance and compliance without pressure. *Psychological Reports, 108*(1), 281–289.

Gneezy, U., & Rustichini, A. (2000). Pay enough or don't pay at all. *The Quarterly Journal of Economics, 115*(3), 791–810.

Gneezy, U., Meier, S., & Rey-Biel, P. (2011). When and why incentives (don't) work to modify behavior. *Journal of Economic Perspectives, 25*(4), 191–210.

Guay, F. (2022). Applying self-determination theory to education: regulations types, psychological needs, and autonomy supporting behaviors. *Canadian Journal of School Psychology, 37*(1), 75–92.

Guay, F., Morin, A. J., Litalien, D., Howard, J. L., & Gilbert, W. (2021). Trajectories of self-determined motivation during the secondary school: A growth mixture analysis. *Journal of Educational Psychology, 113*(2), 390.

Hall, R. V., Lund, D., & Jackson, D. (1968). Effects of teacher attention on study behavior 1. *Journal of Applied Behavior Analysis, 1*(1), 1–12.

Kelley, H. H. (1973). The processes of causal attribution. *American Psychologist*, *28*(2), 107.

Kim, J., McIntosh, K., Mercer, S. H., & Nese, R. N. T. (2018). Longitudinal associations between SWPBIS fidelity of implementation and behavior and academic outcomes. *Behavioral Disorders*, 43, 357–369.

Kohn, A. (1993/1999/2018). *Punished by Rewards: The trouble with gold stars, incentive plans, A's, praise, and other bribes*. United States: Houghton Mifflin Company.

Kong, Y. (2009). A brief discussion on motivation and ways to motivate students in English language learning. *International Education Studies*, *2*(2), 145–149.

Kowalewicz, E. A., & Coffee, G. (2014). Mystery motivator: A Tier 1 classroom behavioral intervention. *School Psychology Quarterly*, *29*(2), 138.

Lassen, S. R., Steele, M. M., & Sailor, W. (2006). The relationship of school-wide positive behavior support to academic achievement in an urban middle school. *Psychology in the Schools*, *43*(6), 701–712.

Lepper, M. R., Greene, D., & Nisbett, R. E. (1973). Undermining children's intrinsic interest with extrinsic reward: A test of the "overjustification" hypothesis. *Journal of Personality and Social Psychology*, *28*(1), 129.

Liu, J. (2004). Childhood externalizing behavior: Theory and implications. *Journal of Child and Adolescent Psychiatric Nursing*, *17*(3), 93–103.

Maggin, D. M., Chafouleas, S. M., Goddard, K. M., & Johnson, A. H. (2011). A systematic evaluation of token economies as a classroom management tool for students with challenging behavior. *Journal of School Psychology*, *49*(5), 529–554.

Maggin, D.l M., Johnson, A. H., Chafouleas, S. M., Ruberto, L. M., & Berggren, M. (2012). A systematic evidence review of school-based group contingency interventions for students with challenging behavior. *Journal of School Psychology*, *50*, 625–654.

Northup, J., George, T., Jones, K., Broussard, C., & Vollmer, T. R. (1996). A comparison of reinforcer assessment methods: The utility of verbal and pictorial choice procedures. *Journal of Applied Behavior Analysis*, *29*(2), 201–212.

O'Connor, K. M., & Hayes, B. (2020). How effective are targeted interventions for externalizing behavior when delivered in primary schools?. *International Journal of School & Educational Psychology*, *8*(3), 161–173.

Reeve, J. (2012). A self-determination theory perspective on student engagement. In S. L., Christenson , A. L., Reschly , & C., Wylie (Eds.), *Handbook of Research on Student Engagement* (pp. 149–172). Boston, MA: Springer

Reiss, S., & Sushinsky, L. W. (1975). Overjustification, competing responses, and the acquisition of intrinsic interest. *Journal of Personality and Social Psychology*, *31*(6), 1116.

Reiss, S. (2005). Extrinsic and intrinsic motivation at 30: Unresolved scientific issues. *The Behavior Analyst*, *28*, 1–14.

Riden, B. S., Kumm, S., & Maggin, D. M. (2022). Evidence-based behavior management strategies for students with or at risk of EBD: A mega review of the literature. *Remedial and Special Education*, *43*(4), 255–269.

Ryan, R. M., & Deci, E. L. (2000). Intrinsic and extrinsic motivations: Classic definitions and new directions. *Contemporary Educational Psychology, 25,* 65–67.

Ryan, R. M., Donald, J. N., & Bradshaw, E. L. (2021). Mindfulness and motivation: a process view using self-determination theory. *Current Directions in Psychological Science, 30*(4), 300–306.

Samek, D. R., & Hicks, B. M. (2014). Externalizing disorders and environmental risk: Mechanisms of gene-environment interplay and strategies for intervention. *Clinical Practice, 11*(5), 537.

Serin, H. (2018). The use of extrinsic and intrinsic motivations to enhance student achievement in educational settings. *International Journal of Social Sciences & Educational Studies, 5*(1), 191–194.

Simmons, J. T., & Wasik, B. H. (1973). Use of small group contingencies and special activity times to manage behavior in a first-grade classroom. *Journal of School Psychology, 11*(3), 228–238.

Smith, S., Barajas, K., Ellis, B., Moore, C., McCauley, S., & Reichow, B. (2021). A meta-analytic review of randomized controlled trials of the good behavior game. *Behavior Modification, 45*(4), 641–666.

Taylor, G., Jungert, T., Mageau, G. A., Schattke, K., Dedic, H., Rosenfield, S., & Koestner, R. (2014). A self-determination theory approach to predicting school achievement over time: The unique role of intrinsic motivation. *Contemporary Educational Psychology, 39*(4), 342–358.

Tian, Y., Fang, Y., & Li, J. (2018). The effect of metacognitive knowledge on mathematics performance in self-regulated learning framework—multiple mediation of self-efficacy and motivation. *Frontiers in Psychology, 9,* 2518.

Walker, H. M., & Hops, H. (1976). Use of normative peer data as a standard for evaluating classroom treatment effects *Journal of Applied Behavior Analysis, 9*(2), 159–168.

Wilson, L. M. & Corpus, D. A. (2001). The effects of reward systems on academic performance. *Middle School Journal, 33*(1), 56–60.

Workman, E. A., & Williams, R. L. (1980). Effects of extrinsic rewards on intrinsic motivation in the classroom. *Journal of School Psychology, 18*(2), 141–147.

Zimmerman, B. J. (1985). The development of "intrinsic" motivation: A social learning analysis. *Annals of Child Development, 2*(1), 117–160.

14 Internalizing Problems

*Avalon S. Moore, Alixandra Wilens, and
Brian A. Zaboski*

Internalizing disorders – including depressive disorders, anxiety disorders, and obsessive-compulsive and related disorders – are common among children and adolescents, ranking among the most damaging causes of disability-adjusted life years lost from fourth grade through postsecondary school (Lew & Xian, 2019; Olivier et al., 2020; World Health Organization, 2021). Nevertheless, less than half (45%) of school-aged children in the United States (U.S.) with a diagnosis receive critical mental health interventions (Green et al., 2013). Consequently, students experience low self-worth, decrements in information processing, poor task mastery compliance, impaired problem-solving strategies, and decreased quality of life (Fredricks et al., 2004; Schrack et al., 2021; Zaboski et al., 2019).

Our understanding of internalizing disorders informs practitioners' ability to address such problems in schools. Thus, we intend to examine two claims related to etiology and intervention for internalizing disorders. First, the contention that depression is caused by a neurochemical imbalance, the veracity of which can yield greater understanding of the impact and place of antidepressants in school-based interventions. Second, the argument that cognitive-behavioral therapy (CBT) with exposure therapy is unethical. Through examining these debates, school psychologists can be better informed on the empirical and theoretical status of common interventions for school children experiencing internalizing problems.

Examining the Claims

Claim 1: Clinical Depression Is Caused by a Chemical Imbalance in the Brain

The neurotransmitter serotonin is involved in autonomic functioning, hormone production, motor skills, cognition, and emotional processing (Zhou et al., 2007). By the 1960s, some researchers believed that the imbalance of serotonin levels in the brain was the singular cause of depression (Coppen, 1967). By the late 1980s to early 1990s, second-generation

DOI: 10.4324/9781003266181-19

antidepressants, also known as selective serotonin reuptake inhibitors (SSRIs), became a first-line psychiatric treatment for patients suffering from depression and continue to be some of the most widely used prescription drugs (Yohn et al., 2017). Early research, the efficacy of SSRIs, and pharmaceutical advertisements have helped perpetuate misunderstandings like *depression is a brain disease, depression is only amenable by medication,* and *school-based interventions cannot address the effects of depression.*

SSRIs and Chemical Imbalances

Proponents of the chemical imbalance theory cite select research that SSRIs modify serotonin levels in the brain (Moncrieff et al., 2022). The 5-hydroxytryptamine (5-HT) deficiency theory of depression, better known as the chemical imbalance theory, began in the 1950s when a drug to combat tuberculosis unexpectedly showed improvement in depressive symptoms for tuberculosis patients (Jacobsen et al., 2012). Since this discovery, second-generation antidepressants (SSRIs) have become the most used prescription medication to treat depression for both children and adults (Yohn et al., 2017).

SSRIs are prescribed to inhibit serotonin transporter proteins from carrying serotonin from the synaptic cleft back into the presynaptic neuron; this process increases the production and overall activity of serotonin in the brain (Ang et al., 2022). Historically, the pharmaceutical industry has invested substantially in advertising and marketing these drugs to not only psychiatrists and other physicians, but to the public (Casey, 2013). These neurochemical effects, combined with the effectiveness of SSRIs and keen pharmaceutical advertising, seem to explain survey results that more than 80% of samples believe that depression is caused by a chemical imbalance in the brain (Pilkington et al., 2013). Since the discovery of SSRIs in the late 1980s/early 1990s, the percentage of patients taking antidepressants has increased by 64% from 1999 to 2014 (Pratt, 2017). Currently, roughly 13% of the current U.S. population over 12 years old takes an antidepressant (Pescosolido, 2013; Pratt, 2017).

Neurobiological Links between Serotonin and Behavior

5-HT, more commonly referred to as serotonin, is a neurotransmitter obtained from an essential amino acid called tryptophan (Maes et al., 2011). The synthesis of serotonin in the brain relies heavily on the bioavailability of tryptophan in the plasma (Fernstrom, 1983). The process of 5-HT synthesis begins when tryptophan is brought into the serotonergic neurons after entering the brain, then hydroxylation to 5-hydroxytryptophan begins by the enzyme, tryptophan hydroxylase; lastly, because this enzyme is not usually saturated by its substrate, the synthesis of 5-HT is determined by changes in the tryptophan's availability and activity (Fernstrom et al., 1976; Maes et al., 2011; Moir & Eccleston, 1968). This process led some early scientists to believe that depression is caused by lowered plasma tryptophan (lowered serotonin), and that the treatment for this deficiency is to increase these serotonin levels in the brain.

Additional evidence that depression has a neurochemical basis originates from tryptophan depletion, a popular mechanism for understanding the brain's serotonergic systems (Bell et al., 2001; Cowen & Browning, 2015). Tryptophan depletion decreases serotonin synthesis and release through the reduction of plasma tryptophan, an amino acid necessary for the synthesis of serotonin (Bell et al., 2001). In one study, short-term depletion of plasma tryptophan resulted in a relapse of depressive symptoms for individuals in remission from major depressive disorder (Bremner et al., 1997). Furthermore, lower levels of plasma tryptophan have been found in patients with severe forms of depressive symptoms (Cowen & Browning, 2015). By contrast, tryptophan supplementation can lead to decreased levels of combativeness and heightened levels of agreeableness (Young, 2013).

Do SSRIs Really Correct Chemical Imbalances?

Although SSRIs can be efficacious in the treatment of depression for some individuals, this does not demonstrate that depression is caused by a serotonin imbalance. The evidence on tryptophan depletion is dated, has small sample sizes, and methodological confounds (Fusar-Poli et al., 2006; Ruhé et al., 2007). Additionally, a major problem with the argument that depression is caused by a serotonin imbalance is that when someone takes an SSRI, their serotonin levels immediately increase; however, improvement takes around 8 weeks to be effective (Leuchter et al., 2009). Thus, although the "chemical imbalance" is immediately rectified by the drug, the depression is not.

The onset of depression has also been repeatedly shown to be due to several factors beyond biochemistry, including family history, adverse life events, socioeconomic status, gender, hopelessness/helplessness, and perception of self-worth (Beardslee & Gladstone, 2001). School psychologists also recognize through cognitive-behavioral models that depression involves the association between thoughts, feelings, and behaviors that maintain – and help to mitigate – depression (Purvis et al., 2021). For example, in children and adolescents, one of the biggest predictive factors for depression is an accumulation of adverse experiences that lead to depression, increased risk-taking behavior, and problematic academic performance (Burns et al., 2002). The most common adversity that leads to the onset of depression for school-aged children is the grief one experiences after loss (Maughan & McCarthy, 1997); however, loss does not inevitably entail depression (Burns et al., 2002).

How Strong Are the Neurobiological Links between Serotonin and Behavior?

Recent studies in plasma serotonin, metabolites, genetics, and gene-stress interaction show no subsequent relationship between depressive symptoms and serotonin activity; while other studies have found no evidence of lowered serotonin activity in patients who suffer from depression compared to controls (Moncrieff et al., 2022). Other findings suggest the lack of sufficient evidence for any biomarkers as causal predictors of major depressive disorder as well as the relapse or recurrence of depressive symptoms (Kennis et al., 2020). Thus, many psychiatrists have referred to the chemical imbalance theory of depression as an *urban legend* creating an *over-medicalized society* (Lacasse & Leo, 2005; Pies, 2011; however, see Ang, et al., 2022 for a related discussion that explores psychiatry's involvement in perpetuating the serotonin theory of depression).

The negative effects of SSRIs are often overlooked and ignored by pharmaceutical companies, while the benefits are magnified (Dubicka & Goodyer, 2005). This asymmetry of reporting influences perceptions and lifelong reliance on these drugs with insufficient evidence of the chemical imbalance theory to justify their prolonged use and side effects (Eveleigh et al., 2019; Maund et al., 2019; Moncrieff et al., 2022). Consequently, while children are often prescribed SSRIs, fluoxetine and escitalopram are the only SSRIs that are FDA-approved and recommended for children with depression, and psychotherapy remains a first-line intervention (Dubicka & Goodyer, 2005; Dwyer & Bloch, 2019). Thus, despite the use of SSRIs and the public's view that they simply remediate the root cause of depression, CBT – in combination with medication only for treatment-refractory cases – continues to be the preferred method for the treatment of depression in children and adolescents (Bernaras et al., 2019), signifying that depression and its treatment are more complex than a chemical imbalance.

Claim 2: Exposure Therapy for Anxiety, OCD, and Trauma Is Unethical and Impractical

Exposure therapy, often used as part of CBT, is a technique in which clients repeatedly approach fear-inducing stimuli, often gradually, to reduce fear reactions through extinction learning (Craske et al., 2014). Central to arguments against exposure therapy is the ostensible harm it causes. In the *New York Times*, exposure therapy was famously dubbed the "cruelest cure" (Slater, 2003) and described by some psychotherapists as "torture, plain and simple." A survey of 255 trauma experts indicated that barriers for imaginal exposures, such as fears of symptom exacerbation or therapy drop-out, were highest relative to other trauma interventions (e.g., medication, supportive counseling; Leahy, 2007; van Minnen et al., 2010). Moreover, imaginal exposure for trauma-related disorders has been found to reliably exacerbate symptoms in some patients (Foa et al., 2002) – a direct consequence and intent of exposure therapy (Abramowitz et al., 2019).

The intentional harm that exposure causes – higher anxiety and symptom exacerbation – is viewed as intolerable to patients. In another study, over 600 therapists completed the *Therapist Beliefs about Exposure Scale,* and they reported the highest mean score for the item "most clients have difficulty tolerating the distress exposure therapy evokes" (Deacon et al., 2013). A systematic review of the dropout rate for exposure therapy is estimated to be around 19% (Ong et al., 2016), and outside of randomized clinical trials, real-world drop-out rates are likely higher, especially for trauma-related concerns (Najavits, 2015).

Societal Pushback for Exposure

Some arguments against exposure highlight the negative perception of eliciting anxiousness in a society that values avoiding or mitigating anxiety quickly. For example, on college campuses, surveys indicate that half of professors have chosen to use trigger warnings, statements that warn students that the course might expose them to graphic or emotionally challenging content (Kamenetz, 2016). Trigger warnings, safe spaces, and anti-anxiety messages are so integrated into our culture that intentionally causing anxiety seems anathema to the psychotherapist's role as a healer (Anderson, 2021; Bram & Björgvinsson, 2004).

Because exposure therapy sessions are often conducted outside the office (Abramowitz et al., 2019), perception matters even to experts. In a survey of 230 practitioners who treat anxiety in children and adolescents, 47% of respondents affirmed that parental perceptions were a treatment barrier (Reid et al., 2017). Moreover, an anonymous survey of 277 experienced exposure therapists supports the contention that societal views of exposure and response prevention are not trivial. One therapist was even reported to a licensing board for teaching a student the principles of exposure and response prevention for sexual and harm-related thoughts. Furthermore, conference presenters occasionally receive negative reactions from non-expert audiences, and therapists have reported interactions with law enforcement (Schneider et al., 2020).

Training and Session Lengths

Empirically supported treatments are generally related to a practitioner's theoretical orientation (e.g., cognitive-behavioral, humanistic, psychodynamic), and it becomes more unlikely to obtain training outside of these areas if one has never been introduced to them (Karekla et al., 2004). Indeed, outside of programs that offer exposure therapy training, supervision can be difficult to find. Forty-eight percent of therapists reported that lack of training served as a barrier to implementing exposure and response prevention with children and adolescents (Reid et al., 2017). Many practitioners also believe that exposure therapy would be a poor fit for their practice. As the habituation model of anxiety expects a natural decrease in anxiety within and between sessions (Benito & Walther, 2015), many professionals believe that 60–90 minute sessions would prohibit the technique in outpatient and school-based settings that require efficient service delivery.

Does Exposure Therapy Really Cause Intolerable Harm?

For several decades, the myth that exposure therapy causes harm has permeated therapeutic circles (Olatunji et al., 2009), but decades of research have belied this. Although practitioners working with adults and children have concerns about harm (Olatunji et al., 2009; Reid et al., 2017), these concerns rarely materialize. Although anxiety can increase following exposures (Foa et al., 2002), opponents rarely mention that these increases tend to be transient. Moreover, careful examination of exposure therapy's tolerability across the domains of symptom exacerbation and patient preferences also reveals low risk (Olatunji et al., 2009). For instance, 94% of participants reported positive effects of intensive forms of exposure-based treatment (e.g., 3x/week), with a low mean intensity of side effects (Heinig et al., 2022). Although clients may report not liking exposures, they generally rate the usefulness of the intervention highly (Cox et al., 1994). This is consistent with qualitative work in group therapy formats – higher short-term anxiety may be offset by treatment gains and the careful use of gradual challenges to avoid panic-like symptoms (Huynh et al., 2022).

Exposure therapy does not increase drop-out relative to other therapies. A systematic review of randomized controlled trials indicated a weighted drop-out rate of 15%, similar to other cognitive-behavioral techniques (Ong et al., 2016). In one of the more complex applications of exposure therapy – trauma – attrition is also similar (Hembree et al., 2003). Although clinicians often attribute dropout to clients' inability to tolerate exposures, the strongest predictor for attrition is often a variable unrelated to severity or distress (Eftekhari et al., 2020). While opponents of exposure therapy are correct that randomized clinical trials tend to underestimate dropout rates from exposure therapy (Najavits, 2015), they have not demonstrated that exposure therapy influences dropout more than any other cognitive-behavioral interventions.

How Much Societal Pushback Is There Really for Exposure Therapy?

Experts in exposure therapy recognize that it has an image problem. Consequently, some surveys have suggested that clinicians prefer describing it with less threatening language, like Supported Approach of Feared Experiences-Cognitive Behavioral Therapy (SAFE-CBT; Becker-Haimes et al., 2022). Though it may sound anxiety-provoking, exposure therapy is recommended by numerous national and international organizations as a first-line intervention for anxiety disorders, posttraumatic stress disorder, and obsessive-compulsive disorder (OCD; e.g., American Psychological Association, 2006; Anxiety and Depression Association of America, 2015; The International OCD Foundation, n.d.)

Serious negative consequences are often cited by opponents, but they are "rare and primarily represent unintended secondary consequences of OCD or limited understanding of the process and rationale behind [exposure and response prevention]" (Schneider et al., 2020, p. 427). Professional Training also mitigates these, decreasing the likelihood of high intensity reactions, improving overall knowledge, and engendering more positive attitudes toward exposure therapy (Farrell et al., 2013; Trivasse et al., 2020). Although there are some cases of litigation, no evidence suggests litigation is more common than with any other technique (Richard & Gloster, 2007; Schneider et al., 2020). This is likely because exposure therapy provokes a response that clients are already experiencing within the context of therapeutic collaboration, rapport, and consent (Olatunji et al., 2009).

Training Opportunities and Session Length

Exposure therapy can be difficult to implement in schools without guidance, and practitioners are consistently concerned about the amount of expertise required. (Olatunji et al., 2009; Reid et al., 2017). Nevertheless, excellent resources are available from the International OCD Foundation's training institute (*The International OCD Foundation*, n.d.), books (Abramowitz et al., 2019; Reid et al., 2021) and primer articles for school applications (Zaboski, 2020). Such training addresses the myth that exposure therapy requires vast amounts of session time. That is, contemporary theories (e.g., inhibitory learning theory) suggest that shorter sessions of exposure therapy can be effective as well (Craske et al., 2014).

Summary and Conclusion

The prevalence of internalizing disorders is substantial (Hall & Wolke, 2012; Letcher et al., 2009; O'Connor et al., 2011). The need to understand the etiology of mental illnesses and to implement efficacious, effective, and efficient interventions to address them could not be more central to school psychology research and practice. For adolescents, depressive, anxiety, and OCDs have become a preeminent risk factor for emotional disengagement spanning across all socioeconomic and cultural backgrounds (Olivier et al., 2020). Myths and misconceptions notwithstanding, depression is caused by a confluence of biochemical, psychological, and socioeconomic factors that complicate the overly simplistic chemical imbalance theory. Moreover, far from the "cruelest cure," exposure therapy is a safe and effective treatment for many internalizing disorders in children and adolescents. Pseudoscientific claims about internalizing disorders risk perpetuating stereotypes about mental illness and interfere with evidence-based care in schools. As practitioners, it is our job not only to understand the mechanisms that underlie internalizing disorders, but also to correct misconceptions and foster skepticism against pseudoscientific claims.

References

Abramowitz, J. S., Deacon, B. J., & Whiteside, S. P. (2019). *Exposure therapy for anxiety: Principles and practice*. Guilford Publications.

American Psychological Association. (2006). Beyond worry: How psychologists help with anxiety disorders. https://www.apa.org/topics/anxiety/disorders

Anxiety and Depression Association of America. (2015, September 15). Clinical practice review for social anxiety disorder. https://adaa.org/resources-professionals/clinical-practice-review-social-anxiety

Anderson, D. (2021). An epistemological conception of safe spaces. *Social Epistemology*, *35*(3), 285–311.

Ang, B., Horowitz, M., & Moncrieff, J. (2022). Is the chemical imbalance an 'urban legend'? An exploration of the status of the serotonin theory of depression in the scientific literature. *SSM – Mental Health*, *2*, Article 100098. 10.1016/j.ssmmh.2022.100098

Beardslee, W. R., & Gladstone, T. R. G. (2001). Prevention of childhood depression: Recent findings and future prospects. *Biological Psychiatry*, *49*(12), 1101–1110. 10.1016/S0006-3223(01)01126-X

Becker-Haimes, E. M., Stewart, R. E., & Frank, H. E. (2022). It's all in the name: Why exposure therapy could benefit from a new one. *Current Psychology*, 1–7. 10.1007/s12144-022-03286-6

Bell, C., Abrams, J., & Nutt, D. (2001). Tryptophan depletion and its implications for psychiatry. *British Journal of Psychiatry*, *178*(5), 399–405. 10.1192/bjp.178.5.399

Benito, K. G., & Walther, M. (2015). Therapeutic process during exposure: Habituation model. *Journal of Obsessive-Compulsive and Related Disorders, 6*, 147–157. 10.1016/j.jocrd.2015.01.006

Bernaras, E., Jaureguizar, J., & Garaigordobil, M. (2019). Child and adolescent depression: A review of theories, evaluation instruments, prevention programs, and treatments. *Frontiers in Psychology, 10*. https://www.frontiersin.org/articles/10.3389/fpsyg.2019.00543

Bram, A., & Björgvinsson, T. (2004). A psychodynamic clinician's foray into cognitive-behavioral therapy utilizing exposure-response prevention for obsessive-compulsive disorder. *American Journal of Psychotherapy, 58*(3), 304–320. 10.1176/appi.psychotherapy.2004.58.3.304

Bremner, J. D., Innis, R. B., Salomon, R. M., Staib, L. H., Ng, C. K., Miller, H. L., Bronen, R. A., Krystal, J. H., Duncan, J., Rich, D., Price, L. H., Malison, R., Dey, H., Soufer, R., & Charney, D. S. (1997). Positron emission tomography measurement of cerebral metabolic correlates of tryptophan depletion—Induced depressive relapse. *Archives of General Psychiatry, 54*(4), 364–374. 10.1001/archpsyc.1997.01830160092012

Burns, J. M., Andrews, G., & Szabo, M. (2002). Depression in young people: What causes it and can we prevent it?. *Medical Journal of Australia, 177*(S7), S93–S96. 10.5694/j.1326-5377.2002.tb04864.x

Casey, D. A. (2013). Do antidepressant medications work?. *Pharmacy and Therapeutics, 38*(3), 162–163.

Coppen, A. (1967). The biochemistry of affective disorders. *British Journal of Psychiatry, 113*(504), 1237–1264. 10.1192/bjp.113.504.1237

Cowen, P. J., & Browning, M. (2015). What has serotonin to do with depression?. *World Psychiatry, 14*(2), 158–160. 10.1002/wps.20229

Cox, B. J., Fergus, K. D., & Swinson, R. P. (1994). Patient satisfaction with behavioral treatments for panic disorder with agoraphobia. *Journal of Anxiety Disorders, 8*(3), 193–206.

Craske, M. G., Treanor, M., Conway, C. C., Zbozinek, T., & Vervliet, B. (2014). Maximizing exposure therapy: An inhibitory learning approach. *Behaviour Research and Therapy, 58*, 10–23.

Deacon, B. J., Farrell, N. R., Kemp, J. J., Dixon, L. J., Sy, J. T., Zhang, A. R., & McGrath, P. B. (2013). Assessing therapist reservations about exposure therapy for anxiety disorders: The therapist beliefs about exposure scale. *Journal of Anxiety Disorders, 27*(8), 772–780. 10.1016/j.janxdis.2013.04.006

Dubicka, B., & Goodyer, I. (2005). Should we prescribe antidepressants to children?. *Psychiatric Bulletin, 29*(5), 164–167. 10.1192/pb.29.5.164

Dwyer, J. B., & Bloch, M. H. (2019). Antidepressants for pediatric patients. *Current Psychiatry, 18*(9), 26–42F.

Eftekhari, A., Crowley, J. J., Mackintosh, M.-A., & Rosen, C. S. (2020). Predicting treatment dropout among veterans receiving prolonged exposure therapy. *Psychological Trauma: Theory, Research, Practice, and Policy, 12*, 405–412. 10.1037/tra0000484

Eveleigh, R., Speckens, A., van Weel, C., Oude Voshaar, R., & Lucassen, P. (2019). Patients' attitudes to discontinuing not-indicated long-term antidepressant use:

Barriers and facilitators. *Therapeutic Advances in Psychopharmacology*, 9, 1–9. 10.1177/2045125319872344

Farrell, N. R., Deacon, B. J., Kemp, J. J., Dixon, L. J., & Sy, J. T. (2013). Do negative beliefs about exposure therapy cause its suboptimal delivery? An experimental investigation. *Journal of Anxiety Disorders*, 27(8), 763–771. 10.1016/j.janxdis.2013.03.007

Fernstrom, J. D. (1983). Role of precursor availability in control of monoamine biosynthesis in brain. *Physiological Reviews*, 63(2), 484–546. 10.1152/physrev.1983.63.2.484

Fernstrom, J. D., Hirsch, M. J., & Faller, D. V. (1976). Tryptophan concentrations in rat brain. Failure to correlate with free serum tryptophan or its ratio to the sum of other serum neutral amino acids. *Biochemical Journal*, 160(3), 589–595.

Foa, E. B., Zoellner, L. A., Feeny, N. C., Hembree, E. A., & Alvarez-Conrad, J. (2002). Does imaginal exposure exacerbate PTSD symptoms?. *Journal of Consulting and Clinical Psychology*, 70(4), 1022–1028. 10.1037/0022-006X.70.4.1022

Fredricks, J. A., Blumenfeld, P. C., & Paris, A. H. (2004). School engagement: Potential of the concept, state of the evidence. *Review of Educational Research*, 74(1), 59–109. 10.3102/00346543074001059

Fusar-Poli, P., Allen, P., McGuire, P., Placentino, A., Cortesi, M., & Perez, J. (2006). Neuroimaging and electrophysiological studies of the effects of acute tryptophan depletion: A systematic review of the literature. *Psychopharmacology*, 188(2), 131–143. 10.1007/s00213-006-0493-1

Green, J. G., McLaughlin, K. A., Alegría, M., Costello, E. J., Gruber, M. J., Hoagwood, K., Leaf, P. J., Olin, S., Sampson, N. A., & Kessler, R. C. (2013). School mental health resources and adolescent mental health service use. *Journal of the American Academy of Child & Adolescent Psychiatry*, 52(5), 501–510. 10.1016/j.jaac.2013.03.002

Hall, J., & Wolke, D. (2012). A comparison of prematurity and small for gestational age as risk factors for age 6–13 year emotional problems. *Early Human Development*, 88(10), 797–804. 10.1016/j.earlhumdev.2012.05.005

Heinig, I., Knappe, S., Hoyer, J., Wittchen, H.-U., Richter, J., Arolt, V., Deckert, J., Domschke, K., Hamm, A., Kircher, T., Lueken, U., Margraf, J., Neudeck, P., Rief, W., Straube, B., Ströhle, A., Pauli, P., & Pittig, A. (2022). Effective – and tolerable: Acceptance and side effects of intensified exposure for anxiety disorders. *Behavior Therapy*, 1–41. Advance online publication. 10.1016/j.beth.2022.11.001

Hembree, E. A., Foa, E. B., Dorfan, N. M., Street, G. P., Kowalski, J., & Tu, X. (2003). Do patients drop out prematurely from exposure therapy for PTSD?. *Journal of Traumatic Stress*, 16(6), 555–562. 10.1023/B:JOTS.0000004078.93012.7d

Huynh, A.-T., Gaboury, I., Provencher, M. D., Norton, P. J., & Roberge, P. (2022). Patient acceptability of group transdiagnostic cognitive behavior therapy for the treatment of anxiety disorders in community-based care: A qualitative study. *Clinical Psychologist*, 26(2), 119–128. 10.1080/13284207.2022.2041363

Jacobsen, J. P. R., Medvedev, I. O., & Caron, M. G. (2012). The 5-HT deficiency theory of depression: Perspectives from a naturalistic 5-HT deficiency model, the tryptophan hydroxylase $2^{Arg}439^{His}$ knockin mouse. *Philosophical Transactions of the Royal Society B: Biological Sciences*, *367*(1601), 2444–2459. 10.1098/rstb.2012.0109

Kamenetz, A. (2016, September 7). Half of professors in NPR ed survey have used "trigger warnings." *NPR*. https://www.npr.org/sections/ed/2016/09/07/492979242/half-of-professors-in-npr-ed-survey-have-used-trigger-warnings

Karekla, M., Lundgren, J. D., & Forsyth, J. P. (2004). A survey of graduate training in empirically supported and manualized treatments: A preliminary report. *Cognitive and Behavioral Practice*, *11*(2), 230–242. 10.1016/S1077-7229(04)80034-8

Kennis, M., Gerritsen, L., van Dalen, M., Williams, A., Cuijpers, P., & Bockting, C. (2020). Prospective biomarkers of major depressive disorder: A systematic review and meta-analysis. *Molecular Psychiatry*, *25*(2), 321–338. 10.1038/s41380-019-0585-z

Lacasse, J. R., & Leo, J. (2005). Serotonin and depression: A disconnect between the advertisements and the scientific literature. *PLoS Medicine*, *2*(12), e392. 10.1371/journal.pmed.0020392

Leahy, R. L. (2007). Emotional schemas and self-help: Homework compliance and obsessive-compulsive disorder. *Cognitive and Behavioral Practice*, *14*(3), 297–302. 10.1016/j.cbpra.2006.08.002

Letcher, P., Smart, D., Sanson, A., & Toumbourou, J. W. (2009). Psychosocial precursors and correlates of differing internalizing trajectories from 3 to 15 years. *Social Development*, *18*(3), 618–646. 10.1111/j.1467-9507.2008.00500.x

Leuchter, A. F., Cook, I. A., Marangell, L. B., Gilmer, W. S., Burgoyne, K. S., Howland, R. H., Trivedi, M. H., Zisook, S., Jain, R., McCracken, J. T., Fava, M., Iosifescu, D., & Greenwald, S. (2009). Comparative effectiveness of biomarkers and clinical indicators for predicting outcomes of SSRI treatment in major depressive disorder: Results of the BRITE-MD study. *Psychiatry Research*, *169*(2), 124–131. 10.1016/j.psychres.2009.06.004

Lew, D., & Xian, H. (2019). Identifying distinct latent classes of adverse childhood experiences among us children and their relationship with childhood internalizing disorders. *Child Psychiatry & Human Development*, *50*(4), 668–680. 10.1007/s10578-019-00871-y

Maes, M., Leonard, B. E., Myint, A. M., Kubera, M., & Verkerk, R. (2011). The new '5-HT' hypothesis of depression: Cell-mediated immune activation induces indoleamine 2,3-dioxygenase, which leads to lower plasma tryptophan and an increased synthesis of detrimental tryptophan catabolites (TRYCATs), both of which contribute to the onset of depression. *Progress in Neuro-Psychopharmacology and Biological Psychiatry*, *35*(3), 702–721. 10.1016/j.pnpbp.2010.12.017

Maughan, B., & McCarthy, G. (1997). Childhood adversities and psychosocial disorders. *British Medical Bulletin*, *53*(1), 156–169. 10.1093/oxfordjournals.bmb.a011597

Maund, E., Dewar-Haggart, R., Williams, S., Bowers, H., Geraghty, A. W. A., Leydon, G., May, C., Dawson, S., & Kendrick, T. (2019). Barriers and facilitators to discontinuing antidepressant use: A systematic review and thematic synthesis. *Journal of Affective Disorders, 245*, 38–62. 10.1016/j.jad.2018.10.107

Moir, A. T. B., & Eccleston, D. (1968). The effects of precursor loading in the cerebral metabolism of 5-hydroxyindoles. *Journal of Neurochemistry, 15*(10), 1093–1108. 10.1111/j.1471-4159.1968.tb06827.x

Moncrieff, J., Cooper, R. E., Stockmann, T., Amendola, S., Hengartner, M. P., & Horowitz, M. A. (2022). The serotonin theory of depression: A systematic umbrella review of the evidence. *Molecular Psychiatry*. 10.1038/s41380-022-01661-0

Najavits, L. M. (2015). The problem of dropout from "gold standard" PTSD therapies. *F1000prime Reports, 7*(43), 1–8. 10.12703/P7-43

O'Connor, E. E., Dearing, E., & Collins, B. A. (2011). Teacher-child relationship and behavior problem trajectories in elementary school. *American Educational Research Journal, 48*(1), 120–162. 10.3102/0002831210365008

Olatunji, B. O., Deacon, B. J., & Abramowitz, J. S. (2009). The cruelest cure? Ethical issues in the implementation of exposure-based treatments. *Cognitive and Behavioral Practice, 16*(2), 172–180. 10.1016/j.cbpra.2008.07.003

Olivier, E., Morin, A. J. S., Langlois, J., Tardif-Grenier, K., & Archambault, I. (2020). Internalizing and externalizing behavior problems and student engagement in elementary and secondary school students. *Journal of Youth and Adolescence, 49*(11), 2327–2346. 10.1007/s10964-020-01295-x

Ong, C. W., Clyde, J. W., Bluett, E. J., Levin, M. E., & Twohig, M. P. (2016). Dropout rates in exposure with response prevention for obsessive-compulsive disorder: What do the data really say?. *Journal of Anxiety Disorders, 40*, 8–17. 10.1016/j.janxdis.2016.03.006

Pescosolido, B. A. (2013). The public stigma of mental illness: What do we think; what do we know; what can we prove?. *Journal of Health and Social Behavior, 54*(1), 1–21. 10.1177/0022146512471197

Pies, R. (2011). Psychiatry's new brain-mind and the legend of the "chemical imbalance." *Psychiatric Times*, 2. https://www.psychiatrictimes.com/view/psychiatrys-new-brain-mind-and-legend-chemical-imbalance

Pilkington, P. D., Reavley, N. J., & Jorm, A. F. (2013). The Australian public's beliefs about the causes of depression: Associated factors and changes over 16 years. *Journal of Affective Disorders, 150*(2), 356–362. 10.1016/j.jad.2013.04.019

Pratt, L. A. (2017). Antidepressant use among persons aged 12 and over: United States, 2011–2014. *NCHS Data Brief, 283*, 1–8.

Purvis, L. N., Zaboski, B. A., & Joyce-Beaulieu, D. (2021). Core CBT components: Part I. In D. Joyce-Beaulieu & B. A. Zaboski (Eds.), *Applied cognitive behavioral therapy in schools* (pp. 101–116). Oxford University Press. 10.1093/med-psych/9780197581384.003.0006

Reid, A. M., Bolshakova, M. I., Guzick, A. G., Fernandez, A. G., Striley, C. W., Geffken, G. R., & McNamara, J. P. (2017). Common barriers to the dissemination of exposure therapy for youth with anxiety disorders. *Community Mental Health Journal, 53*(4), 432–437. 10.1007/s10597-017-0108-9

Reid, E. K., Taylor, L. K., Banneyer, K. N., Dominguez, J., Liu, G., Williams, L. L., Zaboski, B. A., Schneider, S. C., & Storch, E. A. (2021). Core CBT components: Part II. In D. Joyce-Beaulieu & B. A. Zaboski (Eds.), *Applied cognitive behavioral therapy in schools* (pp. 117–142). Oxford University Press. 10. 1093/med-psych/9780197581384.003.0007

Richard, D. C., & Gloster, A. T. (2007). Exposure therapy has a public relations problem: A dearth of litigation amid a wealth of concern. In *Handbook of exposure therapies* (pp. 409–425). Elsevier.

Ruhé, H. G., Mason, N. S., & Schene, A. H. (2007). Mood is indirectly related to serotonin, norepinephrine and dopamine levels in humans: A meta-analysis of monoamine depletion studies. *Molecular Psychiatry, 12*(4), 331–359. 10.1038/sj.mp.4001949

Schneider, S. C., Knott, L., Cepeda, S. L., Hana, L. M., McIngvale, E., Goodman, W. K., & Storch, E. A. (2020). Serious negative consequences associated with exposure and response prevention for obsessive-compulsive disorder: A survey of therapist attitudes and experiences. *Depression and Anxiety, 37*(5), 418–428. 10.1002/da.23000

Schrack, A. P., Joyce-Beaulieu, D., MacInnes, J. W., Kranzler, J. H., Zaboski, B. A., & McNamara, J. P. (2021). Intelligence and academic achievement in inpatient adolescents with comorbid anxiety and depression. *Bulletin of the Menninger Clinic, 85*(1), 23–41. 10.1521/bumc.2021.85.1.23

Slater, L. (2003, November 2). The cruelest cure. *The New York Times.* https://www.nytimes.com/2003/11/02/magazine/the-cruelest-cure.html

The International OCD Foundation. (n.d.). Retrieved November 16, 2022, from https://iocdf.org/

Trivasse, H., Webb, T. L., & Waller, G. (2020). A meta-analysis of the effects of training clinicians in exposure therapy on knowledge, attitudes, intentions, and behavior. *Clinical Psychology Review, 80*, 101887. 10.1016/j.cpr.2020. 101887

van Minnen, A., Hendriks, L., & Olff, M. (2010). When do trauma experts choose exposure therapy for PTSD patients? A controlled study of therapist and patient factors. *Behaviour Research and Therapy, 48*(4), 312–320. 10.1016/j.brat. 2009.12.003

World Health Organization. (2021). *Assessing and supporting adolescents' capacity for autonomous decision-making in health care settings: A tool for health-care providers.* World Health Organization. https://apps.who.int/iris/handle/10665/350208

Yohn, C. N., Gergues, M. M., & Samuels, B. A. (2017). The role of 5-HT receptors in depression. *Molecular Brain, 10*(28), 1–12. 10.1186/s13041-017-0306-y

Young, S. N. (2013). The effect of raising and lowering tryptophan levels on human mood and social behaviour. *Philosophical Transactions of the Royal Society B: Biological Sciences, 368*(1615), 20110375. 10.1098/rstb. 2011.0375

Zaboski, B. A. (2020). Exposure therapy for anxiety disorders in schools: Getting started. *Contemporary School Psychology, 1–6.* 10.1007/s40688-020-00301-0

Zaboski, B. A., Gilbert, A., Hamblin, R., Andrews, J., Ramos, A., Nadeau, J. M., & Storch, E. A. (2019). Quality of life in children and adolescents with obsessive-compulsive disorder: The pediatric quality of life enjoyment and satisfaction questionnaire (PQ-LES-Q). *Bulletin of the Menninger Clinic*, *83*(4), 377–397. 10.1521/bumc_2019_83_03

Zhou, M., Engel, K., & Wang, J. (2007). Evidence for significant contribution of a newly identified monoamine transporter (PMAT) to serotonin uptake in the human brain. *Biochemical Pharmacology*, *73*(1), 147–154. 10.1016/j.bcp.2006.09.008

Postscript

School Psychology Practices with Strong Evidence

Sarah J. Conoyer, Stephen Hupp, and Michael I. Axelrod

Now that you're at the end of this book, you may be feeling discouraged about the field of school psychology. Remember, though, that the focus of this book has been to critique (some may say "tattle on") the more controversial aspects of the field. Fortunately, there are many school psychology practices with a strong research base. Thus, we'd like to end on a positive note by tootling on several fantastic resources.

Many school psychologists refer to the What Works Clearinghouse (WWC), a reputable resource that reviews research on educational practices and programs. Established by the Institute of Education Sciences (IES) within the U.S. Department of Education, the WWC website (https://ies.ed.gov/ncee/wwc) houses various products to assist educators in making evidence-informed decisions regarding intervention and curricula supports. The WWC provides rigorous reviews, summarizes findings, and disseminates information to the public.

Practice guides from the WWC are developed by a panel of educators with expertise in a specific domain (i.e., reading, mathematics, and written expression) in conjunction with empirical literature. The goal is to address a variety of strategies that can be adapted for implementation at multiple levels of an intervention framework such as multi-tiered systems of support (WWC, 2022). While these guides do not focus on a specific product or program, the suggested strategies can be used as part of an intervention framework at the universal level by being embedded into core curriculum. The strategies can also be used to support supplemental and intensive intervention based on individual student needs.

The WWC breaks down evidence of effectiveness for practice guides into four main categories: 1) Strong Evidence, 2) Moderate Evidence, 3) Promising Evidence, or less impressively, 4) evidence that at a minimum "demonstrates a rationale for a recommendation" (WWC, 2022, p. 13). These categories are aligned with evidence definitions from the Every Student Succeeds Act (ESSA; WWC, 2022). For example, the Strong

DOI: 10.4324/9781003266181-20

Evidence characterization indicates that these practices meet WWC standards without reservations based on well-designed research with significant positive effects for a minimum of 350 students across at least two educational locations. These levels of evidence are used for both individual intervention programs as well as general practice guides. Table 15.1 represents strategies from the WWC practice guides with Strong Evidence in each academic domain.

The WWC also offers a limited focus on social-emotional learning and behavior-based strategies. For example, the WWC lists 27 additional social-emotional learning and behavior programs, but only 1 meets the criteria for the Strong Evidence characterization at this time – the Good Behavior Game (WWC, 2023).

For a valuable resource focused primarily on psychological disorders and related behaviors, school psychologists can also reference the website for the

Table 15.1 WWC Practice Guides with Strong Evidence

Academic Domain	*Practices for K-12 Learners with Strong Evidence*
Reading	• Increase awareness of segments of speech sounds and connections to letters. • Teach word decoding, word parts analysis, and word recognition. • Build decoding skills with the goal of reading complex multisyllabic words. • Provide fluency-building activities. • Use comprehension-building practices.
Written Expression	• Teach the writing process for various purposes. • Teach writing strategies using the Model-Practice-Reflect cycle.
Mathematics	• Provide systematic instruction to develop understanding of mathematical ideas. • Teach mathematical language. • Use a well-chosen set of concrete and semi-concrete representations. • Teach the use of visual representations. • Use number lines. • Provide instruction on word problems. • Include timed activities. • Assist in monitoring and reflecting on the problem-solving process.
Academic Content and Literacy for English Learners	• Teach academic vocabulary words intensively using variety. • Provide structured opportunities for developing written language skills.

Note: This list was created in 2023 and influenced by several practice guides from the WWC website (https://ies.ed.gov/ncee/wwc/) and is included in the References section. The WWC provides more specific steps and breaks down the strategies based on grade bands.

Society of Clinical Child and Adolescent Psychology (SCCAP, n.d.; https://effectivechildtherapy.org/concerns-symptoms-disorders/) which identifies treatments based on five categories: 1) Works Well, 2) Works, 3) Might Work, 4) Untested, and 5) Tested and Does Not Work. The psychosocial treatments that meet the criteria for Works Well (also called *well-established treatments*) have been shown to be efficacious in rigorous research by at least two research teams. These treatments are identified in Table 15.2.

Table 15.2 Psychosocial Treatments for Youth That Work Well

Disorder/Behavior	*Well-Established Treatments*
Autism Spectrum Disorder	Applied Behavior Analysis
Attention-Deficit/ Hyperactivity Disorder	Behavioral Parent Training
	Behavioral Classroom Management
	Behavioral Peer Interventions
	Organization Training
Schizophrenia	Multimodal Therapy
	Family-Focused Therapy
	Cognitive-Behavioral Therapy for Psychosis
Bipolar Disorders	Family Skill Building Plus Psychoeducation
Depressive Disorders	Cognitive-Behavioral Therapy (adolescents)
	Interpersonal Psychotherapy (adolescents)
Anxiety Disorders	Cognitive-Behavioral Therapy
	Education
	Exposure
	Modeling
Obsessive-Compulsive Disorder	Family-Focused Cognitive-Behavioral Therapy
Posttraumatic Stress Disorder	Trauma-Focused Cognitive-Behavioral Therapy
Disruptive Behavior	Parent Behavior Therapy (children)
	Combined Behavioral, Cognitive, and Family Therapies (adolescents)
Anorexia/Bulimia	Family-Based Treatment
Overweight/Obesity	Behavioral Treatment (children)
Bedwetting	Urine Alarm (children)
	Dry-Bed Training (children)
Poor Sleep	Cognitive-Behavioral Therapy for Insomnia
	Brief Behavioral Therapy
	Behavioral interventions
Substance Use	Cognitive-Behavioral Therapy (adolescents)
	Motivational Enhancement Treatment with CBT (adolescents)
	Family-Based Treatment – Ecological (adolescents)
Self-Harm/Ideation	Dialectical Behavior Therapy (adolescents)

Note: A version of this table was originally published in Hupp & Hupp (2024) and influenced by several pages from the website for the Society of Clinical Child and Adolescent Psychology (SCCAP) and several systematic reviews (see the References section).

Overall, a growing body of evidence supports many practices and treatments that can benefit students developmentally, educationally, emotionally, and socially. In fact, the identification of effective practices makes the use of ineffective practices in school psychology and education all the more troublesome. This book's first chapter offers evidence of school psychology's self-correction crisis, or the discipline's failure to drive dubious practices from the field. Most of the book's dubious topics continue in practice despite research, decades in some cases, rejecting their scientific and applied value. Fortunately, many assessment, instructional, intervention, and prevention practices exist that have strong scientific support and those practices are being emphasized in school psychology training programs and employed by school psychologists every day. Furthermore, school psychology has led education reform efforts to advance the implementation of research-supported practices. Relying on collaborative frameworks to support change, school psychologists are positioned to influence school-based practices that support all students. Yet, knowing what might work is not enough. School psychologists must approach all ideas critically, promote thoughtful analysis, and champion much-needed self-correction.

Additional Useful Resources

Promoting Academic Skills

- Texas Center for Learning Disabilities (www.texasldcenter.org)
- Florida Center for Reading Research (www.fcrr.org)
- The Science of Math (www.thescienceofmath.com)
- National Center on Intensive Intervention (www.intensiveintervention.org)
- Intervention Central (https://www.interventioncentral.org/)
- The IRIS Center (https://iris.peabody.vanderbilt.edu/)
- Evidence-Based Intervention Network (https://education.missouri.edu/ebi/)
- The Meadows Center for Preventing Educational Risk (meadowscenter.org)
- Blueprints for Healthy Youth Development (https://www.blueprintsprograms.org/)

Behavior and Social-Emotional Learning

- National Center on Intensive Intervention (www.intensiveintervention.org Academic)
- Intervention Central (https://www.interventioncentral.org/)
- The IRIS Center (https://iris.peabody.vanderbilt.edu/)

- Evidence-Based Intervention Network (https://education.missouri.edu/ebi/)
- The Meadows Center for Preventing Educational Risk (meadowscenter.org)
- Blueprints for Healthy Youth Development (https://www.blueprints programs.org/)
- Center on Positive Behavioral Intervention Supports (https://www.pbis.org/)
- PBIS World (https://www.pbisworld.com/)
- Collaborative for Academic, Social, and Emotional Learning (https://casel.org/)
- National Center for School Mental Health (https://www.schoolmental health.org/)
- Evidence-Based Practices Resource Center (https://www.samhsa.gov/resource-search/ebp)

References

Hupp, S. & Hupp, V. (2024). Science-based clinical psychology. In J. N. Stea & S. Hupp (Eds.), *Investigating clinical psychology: Pseudoscience, fringe science, and controversies*. Routledge.

Society of Clinical Child and Adolescent Psychology (n.d.). Retrieved from https://effectivechildtherapy.org/concerns-symptoms-disorders/

What Works Clearinghouse, Institute of Education Sciences, U.S. Department of Education (2023, May). Good Behavior Game. https://whatworks.ed.gov

What Works Clearinghouse (2022). What Works Clearinghouse procedures and standards handbook, version 5.0. U.S. Department of Education, Institute of Education Sciences, National Center for Education Evaluation and Regional Assistance (NCEE). This report is available on the What Works Clearinghouse website at https://ies.ed.gov/ncee/wwc/Handbooks.

Practices Guides Used in the Development of Table 15.1.

Foorman, B., Beyler, N., Borradaile, K., Coyne, M., Denton, C. A., Dimino, J., Furgeson, J., Hayes, L., Henke, J., Justice, L., Keating, B., Lewis, W., Sattar, S., Streke, A., Wagner, R., & Wissel, S. (2016). *Foundational skills to support reading for understanding in kindergarten through 3rd grade (NCEE 2016–4008)*. Washington, DC: National Center for Education Evaluation and Regional Assistance (NCEE), Institute of Education Sciences, U.S. Department of Education. Retrieved from the NCEE website: http://whatworks.ed.gov.

Fuchs, L.S., Newman-Gonchar, R., Schumacher, R., Dougherty, B., Bucka, N., Karp, K.S., Woodward, J., Clarke, B., Jordan, N. C., Gersten, R., Jayanthi, M., Keating, B., and Morgan, S. (2021). *Assisting students struggling with mathematics: Intervention in the elementary grades (WWC 2021006)*. Washington, DC: National Center for Education Evaluation and Regional

Assistance (NCEE), Institute of Education Sciences, U.S. Department of Education. Retrieved from http://whatworks.ed.gov/.

Graham, S., Bollinger, A., Booth Olson, C., D'Aoust, C., MacArthur, C., McCutchen, D., & Olinghouse, N. (2012). *Teaching elementary school students to be effective writers: A practice guide (NCEE 2012–4058).* Washington, DC: National Center for Education Evaluation and Regional Assistance, Institute of Education Sciences, U.S. Department of Education. Retrieved from http://ies.ed.gov/ncee/wwc/publications_reviews.aspx#pubsearch.

Graham, S., Bruch, J., Fitzgerald, J., Friedrich, L., Furgeson, J., Greene, K., Kim, J., Lyskawa, J., Olson, C.B., & Smither Wulsin, C. (2016). *Teaching secondary students to write effectively (NCEE 2017–4002).* Washington, DC: National Center for Education Evaluation and Regional Assistance (NCEE), Institute of Education Sciences, U.S. Department of Education. Retrieved from the NCEE website: http://whatworks.ed.gov.

Vaughn, S., Gersten, R., Dimino, J., Taylor, M. J., Newman-Gonchar, R., Krowka, S., Kieffer, M. J., McKeown, M., Reed, D., Sanchez, M., St. Martin, K., Wexler, J., Morgan, S., Yañez, A., & Jayanthi, M. (2022). *Providing reading interventions for students in Grades 4–9 (WWC 2022007).* Washington, DC: National Center for Education Evaluation and Regional Assistance (NCEE), Institute of Education Sciences, U.S. Department of Education. Retrieved from https://whatworks.ed.gov/.

Woodward, J., Beckmann, S., Driscoll, M., Franke, M., Herzig, P., Jitendra, A., Koedinger, K. R., & Ogbuehi, P. (2012). *Improving mathematical problem solving in grades 4 through 8: A practice guide (NCEE 2012-4055).* Washington, DC: National Center for Education Evaluation and Regional Assistance, Institute of Education Sciences, U.S. Department of Education. Retrieved from http://ies.ed.gov/ncee/wwc/publications_reviews.aspx#pubsearch/.

Reviews Used for the Development of Table 15.2

Altman, M., & Wilfley, D. (2015). Evidence update on the treatment of overweight and obesity in children and adolescents. *Journal of Clinical Child and Adolescent Psychology, 44*(4), 521–537. 10.1080/15374416.2014.963854

Brickman, H. M. & Fristad, M. A. (2022). Psychosocial treatments for bipolar disorder in children and adolescents. *Annual Review of Clinical Psychology, 18,* 291–327. 10.1146/annurev-clinpsy-072220-021237

Comer, J.S., Hong, N., Poznanski, B., Silva, K., & Wilson, M. (2019). Evidence base update on the treatment of early childhood anxiety and related problems. *Journal of Clinical Child and Adolescent Psychology, 48*(1), 1–15. 10.1080/15374416.2018.1534208

Datta, N., Matheson, B.E., Citron, K., Van Wye, E.M., & Lock, J.D. (2022). Evidence based update on psychosocial treatments for eating disorders in children and adolescents. *Journal of Clinical Child & Adolescent Psychology, 52*(2), 159–170. DOI: 10.1080/15374416.2022.2109650

Dorsey, S., McLaughlin, K. A., Kerns, S. E. U., Harrison, J. P., Lambert, H. K., Briggs, E. C., Cox, J. R., & Amaya-Jackson, L. (2016). Evidence base update for psychosocial treatments for children and adolescents exposed to traumatic events. *Journal of Clinical Child and Adolescent Psychology*, 46(3), 303–330. 10.1080/15374416.2016.1220309

Evans, S., Owens, J., & Bunford, N. (2014). Evidence-based psychosocial treatments for children and adolescents with attention-deficit/hyperactivity disorder. *Journal of Clinical Child and Adolescent Psychology*, 43(4), 527–551. 10.1080/15374416.2013.850700

Freeman, J., Benito, K., Herren, J., Kemp, J., Sung, J., Georgiadis, C., Arora, A., Walther, M. & Garcia, A. (2018). Evidence base update of psychosocial treatments for pediatric obsessive-compulsive disorder: Evaluating, improving, and transporting what works. *Journal of Clinical Child and Adolescent Psychology*, 47(5), 669–698. 10.1080/15374416.2018.1496443

Fristad, M. A., & MacPherson, H. A. (2014). Evidence-based psychosocial treatments for child and adolescent bipolar spectrum disorders. *Journal of Clinical Child and Adolescent Psychology*, 43(3), 339–355. 10.1080/15374416.2013.822309

Glenn, C. R., Esposito, E. C., Porter, A. C., & Robinson, D. J. (2019). Evidence base update of psychosocial treatments for self-injurious thoughts and behaviors in youth. *Journal of Clinical Child & Adolescent Psychology*, 48(3), 357–392.

Higa-McMillan, C.K., Francis, S.E., Rith-Najarian, L., & Chorpita, B.F. (2016). Evidence base update: 50 Years of research on treatment for child and adolescent anxiety. *Journal of Clinical Child and Adolescent Psychology*, 45(2), 91–113, 10.1080/15374416.2015.1046177

Hogue, A., Henderson, C. E., Becker, S. J., & Knight, D. K. (2018). Evidence base on outpatient behavioral treatments for adolescent substance use, 2014–2017: Outcomes, treatment delivery, and promising horizons. *Journal of Clinical Child and Adolescent Psychology*, 47(4), 499–526. 10.1080/15374416.2018.1466307

Kaminski, J. & Claussen, A. (2017). Evidence based update for psychosocial treatments for disruptive behaviors in children. *Journal of Clinical Child and Adolescent Psychology*, 46(4), 477–499. 10.1080/15374416.2017.1310044

Lecomte, T., Abidi, S., Garcia-Ortega, I., Mian, I., Jackson, K., Jackson, K., & Norman, R. (2017). Canadian treatment guidelines on psychosocial treatment of schizophrenia in children and youth. *The Canadian Journal of Psychiatry*, 62(9), 648–655.

McCart, M. R., Sheidow, A. J., & Jaramillo, J. (2022). Evidence-based update of psychosocial treatments for adolescents with disruptive behavior. *Journal of Clinical Child and Adolescent Psychology (online first publication)*. DOI: 10.1080/15374416.2022.2145566

Shepard, J. A., Poler Jr., J. E., & Grabman, J. H. (2017). Evidence-based psychosocial treatments for pediatric elimination disorders. *Journal of Clinical Child and Adolescent Psychology*, 46(6), 767–797. 10.1080/153784416.2016.1247356

Stoll, R. D., Pina, A. A., & Schleider, J. (2020). Brief, non-pharmacological, interventions for pediatric anxiety: Meta-analysis and evidence base status. *Journal of Clinical Child & Adolescent Psychology*, 49(4), 435–459.

Smith, T., & Iadarola, S. (2015) Evidence base update for autism spectrum disorder, *Journal of Clinical Child & Adolescent Psychology*, 44(6), 897–922. DOI: 10.1080/15374416.2015.1077448

Weersing, V. R., Jeffreys, M., Do, M. C. T., Schwartz, K. T., & Bolano, C. (2017). Evidence base update of psychosocial treatments for child and adolescent depression. *Journal of Clinical Child & Adolescent Psychology*, 46(1), 11–43.

Index